NEVER GIVE UP

D0827383

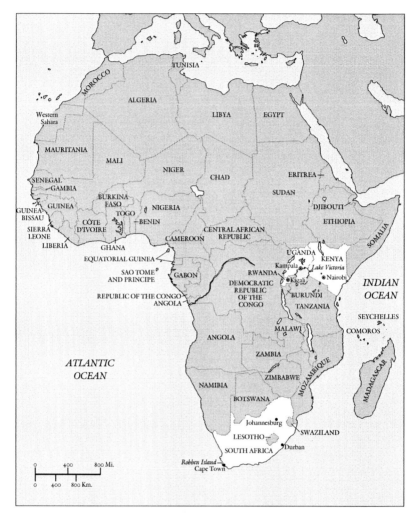

TUNISIA
MOROCCO
ALGERIA
Western
Sahara
LIBYA   EGYPT
MAURITANIA
MALI
NIGER
SENEGAL   CHAD   ERITREA
GAMBIA   SUDAN
GUINEA- GUINEA   BURKINA   DJIBOUTI
BISSAU   FASO   NIGERIA
          CÔTE   TOGO BENIN   ETHIOPIA
SIERRA   D'IVOIRE   CENTRAL AFRICAN
LEONE   CAMEROON REPUBLIC
LIBERIA   GHANA   SOMALIA
         EQUATORIAL GUINEA   UGANDA   KENYA
                                                  Kampala Lake Victoria
         SAO TOME   GABON   RWANDA   Nairobi   INDIAN
         AND PRINCIPE   DEMOCRATIC Kigali   OCEAN
                                        REPUBLIC   BURUNDI
         REPUBLIC OF THE CONGO   OF THE   SEYCHELLES
                   ANGOLA   CONGO   TANZANIA
                                                                       COMOROS
                                        MALAWI
ATLANTIC   ANGOLA
OCEAN   ZAMBIA
                                        ZIMBABWE
                     NAMIBIA
                              BOTSWANA   MOZAMBIQUE
                                                                       MADAGASCAR
                                        Johannesburg
                                        LESOTHO   SWAZILAND
0   400   800 Mi.   SOUTH AFRICA Durban
                              Robben Island
0   400   800 Km.   Cape Town

AFRICA

Never Give Up

VIGNETTES FROM SUB-SAHARAN AFRICA
IN THE AGE OF AIDS

Kevin Winge

SYREN BOOK COMPANY
MINNEAPOLIS

Most Syren Books are available at special quantity discounts
for bulk purchases for sales promotions, premiums, fund-
raising, and educational needs. For details, write

Syren Book Company
Special Sales Department
5120 Cedar Lake Road
Minneapolis, MN 55416

Published by
Syren Book Company
5120 Cedar Lake Road
Minneapolis, MN 55416

Printed in the United States of America on acid-free paper

ISBN-13: 978-0-929636-65-8
ISBN-10: 0-929636-65-1

LCCN 2006926233

Cover design by Kyle G. Hunter
Book design by Wendy Holdman

To order additional copies of this book see the form
at the back of this book or go to www.itascabooks.com

To

Kevin Shores
Birdeen and Delores Winge
John Frey and Jane Letourneau

CONTENTS

PREFACE

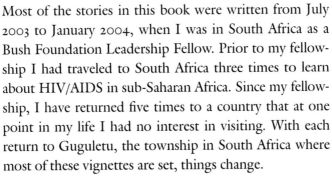

Most of the stories in this book were written from July 2003 to January 2004, when I was in South Africa as a Bush Foundation Leadership Fellow. Prior to my fellowship I had traveled to South Africa three times to learn about HIV/AIDS in sub-Saharan Africa. Since my fellowship, I have returned five times to a country that at one point in my life I had no interest in visiting. With each return to Guguletu, the township in South Africa where most of these vignettes are set, things change.

On my first visit in 2000, the Zwane Community Centre in Guguletu consisted of half a dozen metal cargo containers welded together. Home health care workers, who volunteered their time, met in one corner of the small metal building. Youngsters attending an after-school tutoring program sat on each other's laps. The kitchen consisted of a paraffin burner. Today, visitors to Guguletu see the tall clock tower of the new Zwane Centre long before they actually arrive at the large, modern building that has replaced the shipping containers of a few years ago. The new center, complete with classrooms, community meeting space, offices, and a kitchen that includes stoves, refrigerators, and freezers, has become a hub of township life and is home to programs addressing the seemingly insurmountable issues of lack of education and health care, poverty, violence, and HIV/AIDS.

On a cold Tuesday afternoon in 2002, I was invited to attend an HIV/AIDS support group that had been formed at Zwane. At the first meeting I attended, a dozen women sat in a small circle talking about being HIV-positive. I felt like an eavesdropper on a very private conversation. A participant would occasionally translate what had been said in Xhosa for the benefit of the Western visitors who had joined the group that day. It was depressing. At that time in the townships of South Africa there was little that could be done for these women—except to listen to them. But things change.

That HIV/AIDS support group has continued to meet every Tuesday afternoon. On my most recent visit with the group, nearly 100 participants showed up. Group members still tell their stories and ask each other for advice, but they also share information regarding services and programs that are available for people living with the disease. They report on who is ill and who from the group will go to visit those too sick to come to the meetings. They announce who has died, when the funeral will be, and who from the support group will attend the funeral. From that first small group of women who met a few years earlier, the group has grown and spawned other groups, including a support group for HIV-positive men—something that would have been unheard of in 2002, when many more South African men were in denial about HIV/AIDS than they are today.

Also unimagined in 2002 was the possibility that

someday anti-retroviral medications (ARVs), the drugs that are keeping so many people with HIV/AIDS in the developed world alive, might be available—albeit in very small quantities—to some members of this very support group. Pioneering work done in Haiti by Dr. Paul Farmer and his organization, Partners in Health, along with successful ARV pilot programs by groups such as Médecins Sans Frontières (Doctors Without Borders), have proved that poor, sick people in resource-poor settings can adhere to complicated drug regimens and can thrive—just like privileged people in the West can—if they have access to the same drugs. Each time I go back to the support group meetings, a few more people have qualified for these life-sustaining drugs. But, the overwhelming majority of South Africans living with HIV/AIDS who need these drugs—and need them today—are not getting them.

What happens to some of those people who can't get the medications? On every return visit I make to Guguletu, the cemetery comes perilously closer to being entirely filled with graves. Indeed, by American standards, the cemetery is already full. Now, the gravediggers walk through the cemetery looking for the smallest patch of unused ground to bury one more body.

Some things do not change.

South African president, Thabo Mbeki, who has done many positive things for his country since being elected after Nelson Mandela, has—on the issue of ARVs in specific and HIV/AIDS in general—been out to lunch.

I was at the International AIDS Conference in Durban, South Africa, in July of 2000 and listened to President

Mbkei as he made a causal connection between poverty and AIDS. The next day at the conference a doctor showed a slide of the human immune-deficiency virus (HIV) and, to the thunderous applause of the delegates, announced that this virus—not poverty—causes AIDS.

Despite decades of research on the disease, President Mbeki has continued to dispute established science. He claims there is no link between HIV and AIDS. He says that he personally has never known anyone who died of AIDS, or known anyone who was even HIV-positive. He appointed Manto Tshabalala-Msimang as South Africa's health minister. Dr. Msimang is best known for her comments urging people with HIV/AIDS to eat more garlic and African potatoes rather than take anti-retroviral medications. All of this from the president of the nation that has more people living with HIV/AIDS than any other country on the planet.

♦

Fortunately, often when there is a leadership vacuum, someone appears to fill that void. And at times, leaders arise from the most unexpected places.

As a young man, Zackie Achmat fought against apartheid and was jailed. He worked occasionally as a sex worker. He became a gay activist. He tested positive for HIV. In 1998, with a few others, Mr. Achmat formed the Treatment Action Campaign (TAC) and began advocating for the treatment of all people living with HIV/AIDS in his country. He took on the pharmaceutical companies and sued the South African government in a case that resulted in the Health Ministry having to provide pregnant

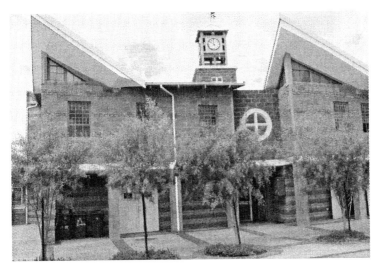

The new Zwane Community Centre in Guguletu: a physical sign of hope in the townships.

women with Nevirapine, a drug that prevents mother-to-child transmission of HIV.

Zackie Achmat's efforts have resulted in international recognition for him and TAC. *Time* magazine has named Mr. Achmat as one of its "heroes." He has been nominated for the Nobel Peace Prize. South Africa's *Globe and Mail* says that Mr. Achmat has "emerged as the greatest figure of moral authority in South Africa since Nelson Mandela." There are reasons to hope for people living with HIV/AIDS in places like South Africa.

I went to South Africa in 2000 because for the first time ever, the International AIDS Conference was being held in a part of the world that was truly suffering the consequences of this plague. In planning the trip with four others from Open Arms of Minnesota, an AIDS service organization based in Minneapolis, we decided to do more than just fly into Durban, attend the conference, and fly back to the United States. We were determined that we would find someone working with HIV/AIDS who could show us what life was like for South Africans with this disease.

For months we delayed making airline reservations as we sent e-mails and letters to North American and African agencies doing work with HIV/AIDS. We left voice messages for people who had volunteered in South Africa or served in the Peace Corps. Our attempts to connect with someone willing to show us their work and help educate us on the issue of HIV/AIDS in sub-Saharan Africa came up short. Finally, one day our travel agent called me and insisted that we make our reservations. The conference was proving to be popular, and the travel agent was concerned that soon all of the flights to Durban would be booked.

I explained our dilemma to the agent—that we were delaying our reservations because of a search to find someone to expose us to the reality of HIV/AIDS on the African continent. "For God's sake," the travel agent said through the phone, "why didn't you tell me? I used to do mission work in South Africa and I just returned from Cape Town. I met a Presbyterian minister there who is very concerned about what AIDS is doing in his community. I have his e-mail address."

I quickly sent an e-mail to that Presbyterian minister, Spiwo Xapile, in one last attempt to identify someone who might be willing to meet with us. I was stunned, a few hours later, when I received a response from Reverend Xapile inviting our group to spend a week with him in Guguletu, South Africa, before attending the conference. He would show us the townships, introduce us to people living with the disease, and generally serve as our host for a one-week intensive primer on AIDS in South Africa. Reverend Xapile is the only person who responded to our inquiries. We immediately accepted his offer, booked our tickets, and changed our lives.

I tell people that on a bad day I'm an atheist and on a good day I'm an agnostic. I say that our introduction to a pastor and Guguletu was a serendipitous coincidence, a strange twist of fate. My friends who are believers in a higher power, no matter what kind of a day they're having, say it wasn't a strange twist of fate at all—they call it a twist of faith. However it happened, an international conference and a travel agent's chance meeting with a minister have had a profound impact on more people than we ever thought possible when we were planning that first trip to South Africa in 2000.

♦

South Africa is a long way from New York City, where the vignettes in this book begin.

I became interested in HIV/AIDS in Africa in the late 1990s. I began to read stories in the *New York Times* about steadily increasing rates of HIV infection in places like South Africa. Now, you didn't need to be a doctor or a scientist to figure out at the time that if HIV rates were rapidly increasing and there were few or no education or treatment programs set up in sub-Saharan Africa, then the world was quickly heading for a major crisis. But the statistics weren't what concerned me. I knew from my friends who had died from HIV/AIDS, who were living with HIV/AIDS, and from my work at Open Arms of Minnesota, that the situation wasn't about statistics—it was about people.

I had seen, especially at the start of the epidemic in the United States, people with HIV/AIDS rejected by their families and friends. I helped them pack up their possessions when they lost their jobs and their homes. There was little I could offer my friends when the very faith communities they went to for support, turned them away. Like so many others, I had waited for Ronald Reagan, our president at the time, to publicly utter the words *HIV/AIDS*. And I waited and waited as thousands more in this country got sick and died and President Reagan continued to do nothing because this was a disease that was primarily affecting gay men and drug users.

By the end of the twentieth century, HIV/AIDS in the United States paled in comparison to what was happening in sub-Saharan Africa. As the worst-case predictions for numbers of HIV cases in Africa were exceeded, year after year, where was the outrage? Where were the Act-Up protesters of the 1980s who demanded services for people living with HIV/AIDS in the U.S. at the time? Where was the leadership insisting that we at least pay as much attention to AIDS in Africa as we paid to what Michael Jackson was doing to his face?

AIDS has always been a disease of "the other" or "those people" or "them." In the 1980s in this country, "those people" were gay men. Then "those people" also became African Americans. More and more, "those people" in the United States are now poor as well. Around the world, "those people" now living with HIV/ AIDS are much more likely to be women, and African, Indian, or Chinese.

I was silent for too long at the start of the AIDS epidemic in the U.S. in the 1980s. I saw, too often, how the majority of the people in this country turned their backs on the first people to contract HIV/AIDS here. I know the devastating impact that had on my friends who got sick and died.

It's happening all over again. Only this time it's not gay men in the Village and in the Castro getting sick; it's poor, black people in townships like Guguletu. If we as individuals don't respond to this epidemic—wherever it occurs and whomever it affects—we are no different from all of those who didn't respond when the first people in this country—our sons, brothers, nephews, cousins, partners, and lovers—went from having HIV, to having full-blown AIDS, to dying. We have an obligation to do something in this country and in other parts of the world to address the HIV/AIDS pandemic.

The vignettes that follow are based on my time in Africa and as seen through my very American eyes. Not all of these scenes are overtly about HIV/AIDS. Some are about different issues, some are about everyday life, but all have a subtext of HIV/AIDS. My intent is to increase awareness of the impact this disease is having on people. I hope to personalize an issue that too many of us walk away from because we think it's just too big and there is nothing that any of us can do.

I am tired of the story of this pandemic being told in statistics about HIV infection and AIDS mortality rates. These numbers are paralyzing us. To understand HIV/AIDS in places like Africa and to be moved to act, we must realize that all of these statistics represent real people.

The people sketched with words in this book are real. Whenever possible, I have used their actual names. In some cases, I felt it was important to change their names. The people whose images appear in the photographs are also real. Some are the actual person who is referred to in the vignette, but that is not always the case. I received permission before taking every photo that appears in the following pages. That said, I did not know at the time I snapped these photos that they would one day be included in a book. I have been successful in securing permission from some of the people depicted in these photos to include their image here. With others, I have no idea who the people are, nor where they currently are, nor how to contact them. It is unlikely that all of them are still alive. I accept the criticism of those who think it inappropriate to use photos of vulnerable people—children and sick people—to tell these stories. I know of no more effective way, however, to emphasize that HIV/AIDS is not about statistics.

These vignettes are based on my life experiences, and not solely my experiences in Africa. They are colored by my political views, emotions, frustrations, sadness, anger, and unfailing optimism and hopefulness. They are not unbiased, but they are true.

ACKNOWLEDGMENTS

♦ ───────────────────────────────

One of the many things I have realized through my involvement and work with HIV/AIDS is just how fortunate I am. I have my health, a job I love, a supportive partner, family and friends. And, I have had opportunities.

I am indebted to The Bush Foundation of St. Paul, Minnesota, and The Bush Leadership Fellows Program of the Bush Foundation for supporting my education at the Kennedy School of Government at Harvard University and my work and writing in Africa. Martha Lee and John Archabal of The Bush Foundation were particularly helpful during my time as a Bush Leadership Fellow.

Sue Williamson and Frank Hartmann at Harvard's Kennedy School of Government were more influential in my writing this book than they probably realize.

Cheryl Chute and Pam Mitman provided encouragement on the earliest drafts to keep me writing. Mary Byers provided a critical eye and the editing skills needed for me to finish the book.

Every day I get to go to work for Open Arms of Minnesota, a nonprofit organization that nourishes body, mind, and soul and has a vision of a world in which people won't go hungry. I couldn't work with a more dedicated and talented group of people—the staff, board of directors and volunteers of Open Arms.

In South Africa, I've been fortunate to discover the same kind of people at the Zwane Community Centre in Guguletu. Spiwo and Zethu Xapile welcomed me into their lives from our very first meeting. The people of Guguletu welcomed me in into their community.

I have been very fortunate in my life. I only wish everyone in the world shared the same good fortune.

NEVER GIVE UP

GUGULETU, SOUTH AFRICA, VIA NEW YORK CITY

Had I never gone to New York in 1983, I never would have gone to South Africa twenty years later. The two experiences are linked.

That spur-of-the-moment decision to throw a few items into a suitcase and drive my Toyota Tercel from Minneapolis to New York was, I see now, a straight line to Cape Town, South Africa. It would take nearly two decades for all the dominos of my life to be lined up, but that first domino that started the chain reaction of events that led to Africa was put in place when I arrived in New York on Valentine's Day, 1983.

I was twenty-four. I had my life's savings—$900—rolled into a pair of socks and a newly awarded bachelor's degree in political science tucked into my backpack. I knew that neither the money nor the degree was going to get me very far. I had no prospects in New York. I knew no one there, which wasn't particularly surprising since I had never been to New York before.

My college roommate had put himself through school working as a waiter in the restaurant of a chain hotel. As a perk of the job, he received certificates redeemable for

accommodations at participating hotels around the country. He had accumulated twenty-one free night stays at
the Statler Hotel across from Madison Square Garden in
midtown Manhattan. That was all my roommate needed
to announce that he was moving to New York, and he
thought I should move with him. He hadn't thought
through what he would do when the three weeks of free
accommodations were gone. Neither had I.

At the time I was working in the box office of a theater
in Minneapolis making reservations for people to see performers like Patti LuPone in Shakespeare's *As You Like It*.
The only joy in my job came from placing rude customers
in the worst possible seats. Well, I also took some joy in
occasionally making up a reason why the box office manager should release house seats for people who were excep-
tionally kind and easy to deal with on the phone. Mostly,
though, I lived to go out after work.

I worked the 1:00 to 9:00 p.m. shift, which fit my
nightclub schedule perfectly. Off work at 9:00. A quick
change of clothes. Pick up some friends. At the bar with
a drink in hand by 10:00. Dancing by 10:30. Drunk by
11:30 and in bed—somewhere—by 1:30 in the morning.

Wake up. Sober up. Swear I was never going to go out
again. Back to work at 1:00 in the afternoon. More reservations for Patti LuPone. More crabby customers. A call
from a friend to go clubbing. Back at the bar by 10:00 that
night.

So when my roommate said I should go with him to
New York, when he pointed out that if I was going to
continue nightclubbing that there were more and better
clubs in New York, that if I was going to make a career

out of taking reservations for Broadway stars I may as well do it on Broadway, what could I say?

I quit my job, stored a few boxes in my parents' basement, loaded the car with a couple of suitcases, and headed east. My life savings didn't allow for the luxury of an overnight stay in a motel. Somewhere in Pennsylvania I pulled into a truck stop, parked my car, and immediately fell asleep.

I didn't know much about New York—didn't know anything about New York, really—but I did know that New York City was no place to have a car. My roommate told me about his cousin who had recently left the city and moved upstate. He had talked to his cousin, who had given his permission for me to leave my car at his house. From there I could take the train to Grand Central Station, where I would emerge from underground to begin a new life in a new city.

That was the plan. Get to Kingston, New York. Find the cousin's house. Spend the night there and the next morning board the train for New York. That was the plan. But it didn't work out that way.

When I woke up behind the steering wheel of my car at the Pennsylvania truck stop, flakes of snow were falling. By the time I turned onto the New York Thruway, it was getting darker and snowing heavier.

A couple of inches of snow were already on the ground when my car crunched to a stop in front of the cousin's house.

I kept the car running, headlights on, wipers barely keeping the windshield clear of snow.

I stared out the window at the large, columned white

house—an impressive though slightly rundown Tara—high above the Hudson River.

What had I done? Just days before I had a job and an apartment in a city filled with friends. Now, I was sitting in my car with a few pathetic possessions in the middle of a snowstorm in a podunk town in New York, totally dependent on the kindness of some stranger I was about to meet.

Fortunately, I didn't have time to second-guess my decision to move halfway across the country on a whim. The headlights signaled to the cousin that his unknown guest had arrived. As the cousin was turning on the porch light and opening the huge door of his house, I was turning off my headlights and opening the door of my car.

Before the cousin had a chance to step out of his house and onto the porch, just as I was closing the car door, a horse of a dog came charging out of the house toward me.

"Chip!" the cousin hollered at the dog. "He won't hurt you," the cousin yelled at me.

With a hundred-pound, chocolate-colored Chesapeake Bay retriever escorting me, I walked up the steps of the porch and introduced myself to the cousin, John.

We quickly entered the house and closed the door on the intensifying winter storm. The foyer of John's house was larger than the apartment I had given up in Minneapolis. I didn't get a tour of the mammoth house that evening. John immediately shuttled me into a tiny study off the foyer—a little room with just enough space for a sofa, a chair, and a bar.

The dog, having shaken all the snow from his coat,

circled an electric space heater several times. With a loud exhalation of air, Chip settled on a spot on the wood floor where he would be close to the heat and in our way for the rest of the evening as John and I would have to step over the dog to get to the bar or the bathroom. With an exhalation of breath to match the dog's, I sank into the cushion of the comfortable sofa.

John apologized for keeping the television on, but a major blizzard was expected to hit New York and he was waiting for a weather update. When the weather report aired a few minutes later and predicted a record-breaking snowfall, John switched off the television, turned to me, and suggested I get comfortable. "I don't think you will be going into the city for a few days," he said.

John walked over to the bar and poured me a scotch on the rocks. He poured himself the same, with a splash of soda, and we talked.

We talked that night until I was nearly falling asleep on the sofa.

We talked all the next day as the snow continued to pile higher and higher outside, and we scoured the kitchen for food to eat, since there was no possibility of leaving the house for groceries.

We talked the day after that as the snow finally stopped, but the closed thruway still prevented me from getting to Manhattan.

And we even talked the next day when the freeway re-opened and the trains were running again, but I was having too much fun to leave John's upstate home.

A Valentine's Day blizzard turned what was to have been a one-night stay in the house of a stranger into a four-day experience that cemented one of the greatest friendships of my life.

I would leave upstate, go into the city, check into the Statler, and eventually get a job at a temp agency and find a more permanent place to stay; but every few weeks I would return to John's house upstate or he would come into the city.

John introduced me to his friends in the city and his friends upstate. He expanded my already quite comprehensive knowledge of cocktails. He played Dinah Washington albums on a turntable—a kind of soul music I never heard in my small hometown. He took me hiking in the Catskills and to dinner and the theater in Manhattan. He piqued my interest in international travel with a trip to South America. And, most important, he taught a twenty-four-year-old kid who didn't think he was naive (but who really was) how to maneuver in New York City. John had his friends in the city look out for me. If I screwed up or made a bad decision, John would hear about it and I would soon hear from John. He was the brother I never had and, in retrospect, a guardian angel.

The early 1980s were halcyon days in New York. Everyone, especially me, was living on credit. We didn't know about AIDS then. There was a mysterious disease called GRID, gay-related immune deficiency, hitting San Francisco and New York, but it would be awhile before HIV would be identified and a test for the virus would become available. That's when the bills came due and people began to get sick and others began to get scared. John's watchful eye, his insistence on knowing who I was associating with and what I was doing, kept me healthy. John wasn't so lucky.

Almost certainly, John was HIV-positive when I met him. By the time a test for the virus was developed a few years later, John was already showing signs of being sick.

We met for dinner in Manhattan the night before he was to have his AIDS test. We both assumed what the results would be.

That night we met for dinner—when was it? Sometime in 1985?—was the last night that AIDS would not be a part of my life. Two weeks later John would call to confirm what we both suspected: he was HIV-positive.

An HIV diagnosis in 1985 was a death sentence. John's doctor gave him two years to live. The doctor was off by nearly a decade, but it was still a death sentence.

♦

The last time I saw John he was in a private room in a hospital in the same upstate town where I first met him. He was going in and out of consciousness. When he was coherent he would rub his eyes and say that he had lost his contact lenses because he was having trouble seeing. His doctor said he was going blind.

John had wasted away. At fifty-four, he looked like a frail old man. I sat by the side of his bed, waiting for pneumonia to come.

No one came to see John on that last day I spent in his hospital room. No nurse came to check on him. I sat in silence by the side of his bed for hours, listening to John's labored breathing. After a few hours I started to get anxious. I needed a break. I just needed to get the hell out of that room.

I opened the door of John's room and stepped into the hospital corridor. There on the floor outside of John's room was his lunch, now cold, left there by an orderly too frightened to bring a meal into the room of an AIDS patient.

If that happened today, I would get angry. I would throw a fit. That day I just didn't have the energy. The meal tray on the floor said it all. I stood in the hall, looking out of the window on an August day so hot I could see the heat rising off the tarred parking lot, and sobbed. Although John was still alive, I knew it was over.

♦

I will never forget what John experienced as he went from being HIV-positive to having full-blown AIDS to dying. How some friends and family abandoned him. How his faith deserted him. How he lost his job and his home and filed for bankruptcy. How so few people in this country seemed to give a damn about a bunch of gay guys getting sick and dying.

John left a few items of personal property to me—a set of rose-colored cordials we used to drink Chartreuse and Sambuca out of and some antique copper pots collected in Colombian villages in the 1960s. But I inherited much more from him than these mere possessions.

John's death was a wake-up call for me. I realized that one day I would have to account for what I did, or what I failed to do, during the AIDS epidemic. I don't mean that I would have to account to a higher power. I would have to account to myself.

Would my compassion end with the death of John and other friends who had tested positive and died? Could I live with the hypocrisy of turning my back on others living with HIV/AIDS the way so many in this country turned their backs on John and thousands like him who were the first to be infected with HIV? What difference did it make if someone with HIV/AIDS was gay or black or female or poor or African? Had AIDS taught me nothing?

If I turned my back on AIDS—be it someone living

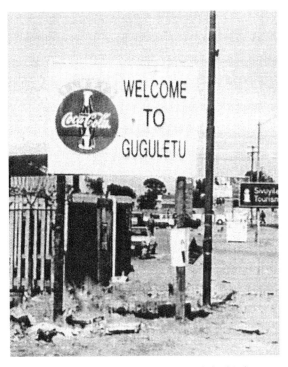

The township of Guguletu has one of the highest rates of HIV infection in the Western Cape of South Africa. A Xhosa word, the name means "our pride."

with the disease down the street from me in Minneapolis, or halfway around the world in African countries—I would be no different from all those who turned their backs on John—and all the others like John—in the 1990s. I knew I couldn't do that and live with myself.

The AIDS pandemic has given me strength and resilience I never knew I had, compassion I didn't know I was capable of.

It has taken me to places in the world I never imagined seeing and introduced me to people I never would have met.

My journey began as an impressionable twenty-four-year-old stuck in a snowstorm in New York. Meeting one person who would become infected with HIV and eventually die of AIDS completely changed my life. HIV/AIDS has since taken me to places I never thought of visiting, let alone living and studying and working in. It brought me back from New York to Minneapolis, Minnesota, and then to Cambridge, Massachusetts, and Guguletu, South Africa. Always back to Guguletu.

These stories—not the material possessions—are my real inheritance from John.

HARVARD

♦ ⎯⎯⎯⎯⎯⎯⎯⎯⎯⎯⎯⎯⎯⎯⎯⎯⎯⎯⎯⎯⎯⎯⎯⎯⎯⎯⎯⎯⎯⎯

The director of graduate programs for the Kennedy School of Government at Harvard University looked at my undergraduate transcript, which was nearly twenty years old and listed more Bs and Cs than As. Then she set the transcript aside and looked at my recent GRE admission test scores, which showed more two-digit numbers than three-digit ones.

"Is your written application brilliant?" the interviewer asked.

"I wouldn't say it's brilliant," was my response.

"Based on these scores, it needs to be brilliant if you're going to get into graduate school at Harvard."

Well, that was that.

I had spent a good deal of money taking a Kaplan course to improve my GRE scores. I had played countless word games on the computer in a lame attempt to increase my verbal score to compensate for my mathematical one. In a similar exercise to improve my analytical score, I repeatedly tried to determine whether a westbound or an eastbound train would arrive at a hypothetical station based on distance and the number of stops each train would make. At the end of the day—at the end of the GRE—my verbal scores were average and my analytical score was lousy. Not as bad as my mathematical score, however, which placed me in the lowest tenth percentile of mathematical ability.

My GRE scores would not gain me admittance to Harvard, nor would my undergraduate transcript. Although I didn't know much about math, I did know that if I plotted my undergraduate grade point average on a graph, it would decrease in direct correlation with increased college partying.

That left only my written application highlighting a leadership example to get me into Harvard. Was the application brilliant? the director asked at the start of the interview.

No.

So, I figured I might as well relax and enjoy the fact that I had come this far. I hadn't just thought about going to Harvard and discounted it as an impossible dream, I had pursued it. I had given it my best shot. I would never have to play the "what if" game. "What if I had applied to Harvard?" I did apply. I did interview. I took a chance, and even though it looked like the outcome wasn't going to go in my favor, I felt great for trying.

Three months later I was at my office when I received an e-mail from Harvard telling me to look for an important fax that had been sent. I rushed to retrieve the fax before anyone else in the office saw it. I got to the fax machine just as the last page was printing.

I grabbed the document and returned to my office and closed the door behind me. I sat down at my desk and read: "Congratulations! I am pleased to offer you admission to the John F. Kennedy School of Government's Program in Public Administration."

Minutes later, another message appeared in my e-mail inbox. I had received a Leadership Fellowship from the Bush Foundation of St. Paul, Minnesota, in the amount of $87,000 to support my studies at Harvard. In addition, upon graduation, the fellowship would sponsor six months of fieldwork in South Africa for me to learn more about the AIDS pandemic in the developing world.

Gaining admittance to Harvard and being awarded a fellowship didn't just happen. It's not as though I opened my e-mail to discover that the universe had decided that my life should take an unanticipated turn. I had thought about graduate school for years and had spent two years— off and on—diligently writing my applications to the Kennedy School and to the Bush Foundation's Fellowship Program.

I knew that this would be the day I would hear from both of them. Still, I was unprepared for the positive responses. I didn't think I fit the profile of someone who gained admission to an Ivy League school, and I certainly didn't think I would be awarded a fellowship in an amount significantly higher than my annual income.

My response to those faxes and e-mails surprised me. I wasn't elated. I was filled with an overwhelming sense of responsibility. I'm not a sentimental person, but my first thoughts were about my family.

None of us in the United States, when we really think about it, are too far removed from the immigrant experience. My great-grandparents came here from Norway in the 1870s. My paternal grandfather lived in a sod house as a homesteader in South Dakota.

My parents' first language was Norwegian, and they were punished in school for not speaking English. The children of farmers rarely went to high school in the 1920s and '30s. Both my father and mother attended one-room schoolhouses and only finished the eighth grade. Most of my older sisters also went to a one-room school-house at the start of their education.

I was the first person in my family to complete a bach-elor's degree, and now I was going to graduate school at Harvard. Of course, I was excited, but that excitement was tempered by all my family had done to make it pos-sible that one day, one of us would have an opportunity like I had just been awarded.

My great-grandparents left Norway, never to see their homeland or their families again, in hopes of creating a better life in America. My grandparents survived depres-sions, locusts, and droughts, all while trying to eke out a living for their families. The one grandfather I remember wouldn't take the bread and wine of communion at his Lutheran church because if he knelt to accept the sacra-ment, the congregation would see the holes in his shoes. His wife, my grandmother who died of cancer just weeks after I was born, might have survived if they could have afforded health insurance.

My father worked as a farmer until a series of heart attacks put an end to that. At forty and with six children to support, my mother went to work as a cook in restau-rants, hospitals, and schools. My teenaged sisters assumed more of the responsibilities at home. Social Security dis-ability payments got us through those lean years.

For generations, my family had worked to build better lives, not just for themselves, but for their children and grandchildren. I would be part of the generation that would benefit from all that they did and from all that they sacrificed.

At Harvard, I met many students whose life experiences were very different than mine. For them, attending Harvard was a birthright. Their parents were alumni, and their parents' parents were alumni. They came from influential and prominent families. But I also discovered I was not alone in my experiences. There were many other students who never imagined that one day they would be attending the oldest university in the nation. Classmates whose parents and grandparents had sacrificed just as much as—if not more than—mine; classmates who, because of socioeconomic status or gender or skin color, didn't have the same opportunities as those who saw attendance at Harvard as their due. I found myself more attracted to this latter part of the student body than the former.

During my year at Harvard I never quite got over the feeling of "Oh my God, I'm actually going to Harvard!" It's thrilling to meet vice presidents, senators, and governors. To have coffee with Pulitzer Prize–winning authors. To take classes from presidential advisers and cabinet members. To have access to one of the best libraries in the world.

The key to Harvard, at least for me, was in not forgetting where I had come from and being very clear about what I wanted to leave with. I wanted to leave Harvard with a greater understanding of how the world operates and an even stronger commitment to change the world.

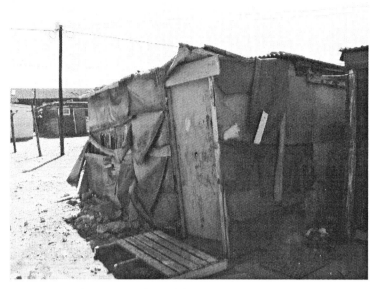

In June of 2003, I graduated from Harvard University in Cambridge, Massachusetts. One month later, I was living in Cape Town, South Africa, and working in Guguletu.

Fortunately, my fellowship from the Bush Foundation allowed me to take all I learned in principle at the Kennedy School and apply it in practice in South Africa.

Nearly a year after I graduated from Harvard and a few months after I returned to the United States from Africa, I had another interview in St. Paul. This one was my final interview with the Bush Foundation. One of the questions they asked me was, "If you had to choose between a master's degree from Harvard, or six months living and working with people living with HIV/AIDS in South Africa, which would you choose?"

The answer was simple.

As great as the year in Cambridge was, for me the real learning was imparted by the people I met and worked with in South Africa, as well as in Uganda and Rwanda—people who, for the most part, are like my parents, grandparents, and great-grandparents: just trying to make a better life for their families under very difficult circumstances.

YOU'VE GOT TO COME IN RIGHT

Noted journalist and CNN's African bureau chief, Charlayne Hunter-Gault, presented a series of lectures titled
"New News Out of Africa" at Harvard University in the
spring of 2003. Over the course of three lectures, one single
comment by Hunter-Gault jumped out and grabbed my
attention.

Hunter-Gault was recalling the start of her career as
a young writer for the *New York Times*. As one of the few
African American reporters working for the newspaper in
the 1960s, she was sent to Harlem to cover a meeting of
the Black Panthers. At the time, the Black Panthers were
feared by many Americans as a radical and violent movement determined to overthrow the U.S. government.
Condemned by politicians and wiretapped by J. Edgar
Hoover's FBI, the Black Panthers had reason to be suspicious of anyone who showed up at a meeting—including
a black woman who was just there to cover the story for
the prestigious *Times*. Denied entrance by a member of
the Black Panthers who was guarding the door, Hunter-
Gault insisted that she be allowed into the meeting. She
explained that she was a cub reporter who could not go
back to her boss without a story. Hunter-Gault, very early

in her career, exhibited the persistence and determination that would make her an accomplished journalist.

It must have been an interesting encounter: two African Americans in the 1960s meeting at a door in Harlem. One was a Black Panther, tired of seeing his movement criticized by the press and instructed to keep reporters out of the meeting. The other was a young reporter determined to go back to her boss with the story she had been sent to get. As anyone who has followed Hunter-Gault's career (be it at the *New York Times,* or public television's *NewsHour with Jim Lehrer,* or now at CNN) could guess, she got into the meeting and got her story. Before relenting to her cajoling, the Black Panther gave the young reporter a piece of advice. He said that he would allow her into the meeting, but he told her, "You've got to come in right."

In telling the story nearly forty years later, Charlayne Hunter-Gault remembers knowing exactly what the man meant. He was admonishing the reporter to set aside preconceived notions—to forget about stories she might have read about the Black Panthers or rumors she might have heard about their activities. He was instructing the reporter to enter the meeting with a clear head and open eyes. To observe. To listen. To be receptive to what she was going to see and hear. To learn. In order to do all of those things, she would have to "come in right."

For three days I had attended Ms. Hunter-Gault's lectures and the follow-up question-and-answer sessions. I sat with a notepad on my lap, ready to record information or new insights into life in South Africa to better prepare myself for my time in the country. It was the story she told about the Black Panthers, the specific quote, that grabbed my attention. It was the best piece of advice I had ever heard about how to enter a new country. I immediately wrote it down on the inside cover of my journal: "You've got to come in right. Charlayne Hunter-Gault, May 15, 2003."

Later, when I arrived in South Africa and found an apartment, got a phone, and opened a bank account, those essentials—my address, telephone number, and bank information—were added to the inside cover of my journal. Every time I opened my journal to find a PIN, I was reminded of the advice handed down from a Black Panther to Charlayne Hunter-Gault to me. "You've got to come in right." My challenge was to figure out the best way to come into South Africa.

♦

We all know the reputation Americans have around the world. We are "the ugly Americans." I arrived in South Africa just months after the United States attacked Iraq in our country's first "pre-emptive" war. George W. Bush's foreign policy did not make it any easier to be an American abroad in 2003.

In traveling internationally, my experience has always been that people in other countries don't hate individual Americans; they hate our policies that have direct and often negative consequences for their nations. During my time on the African continent, I never felt personally attacked because of our government's positions, but being American was often an issue.

A South African nun said to me: "I like you, even though you're American. I'm going to tell people you are my Canadian friend." And she referred to me as her Canadian friend every time I saw her after that. Other Africans told me they would never visit the United States. To do so, they said, would show their support for a nation that had no respect for the developing world.

When I first arrived in Cape Town, I stayed in a small flat owned by the friend of a friend. My friend's friend was eager to rent the apartment, but was hesitant to rent to an American. She only agreed to my staying there when my South African friend assured her that I was not a Bush-supporting, right-wing Republican. Months later, when my friend's friend had become my friend, she confessed to me over a bottle of wine one evening that until she got to know me, she had referred to me as the "fucking American"—as in, "I can't believe I agreed to rent a flat to a fucking American" or "That fucking American who is staying in my flat arrives tomorrow."

I didn't mind the moniker. In fact, I appreciated the fact that my new South African friend told me about her preconceived notions of Americans, and I was grateful to have the opportunity to dispel some of those beliefs. That was, it seemed to me, one way to "come in right" to South Africa: to be proud and open about being an American, and to engage with people in conversations about all aspects—good and bad—of our country. I refused to be like some Americans I met during my time abroad who told me they were embarrassed by our nationality and who always hoped it would not come up in conversations. How could we begin to change other people's impressions of America if we weren't even willing to admit where we came from?

There were times, however, especially when working with some American visitors in the townships, when I understood where the expression "ugly American" comes from. I even understood why some of us are referred to as "fucking Americans."

Very few Americans who visit South Africa spend time in the townships. The majority who travel that far come to enjoy the natural beauty, the beaches, the food and wine of a spectacular and somewhat mysterious country. Any American who goes into the townships, even on one of the brief township tours, is to be commended for making an effort to try to understand a country in its totality.

Those whose primary motivation for traveling to South Africa is to better understand the legacy of apartheid, to see for themselves what life is like in the townships, and to assist efforts to improve the lives of people living with poverty and disease, are deserving of even greater accolades. It is no vacation to spend time with children who have been orphaned by HIV/AIDS or whose families have discarded them because they have mental or physical handicaps. It's no day at the beach walking through hospitals or hospices with bed after bed filled with patients who may be dying in front of your eyes. It isn't fun to talk face-to-face with a young woman who was gang-raped and became infected with HIV, or to discover that the only place a man dying of AIDS has to sleep is in the outhouse behind a cousin's home.

People should be applauded for using their vacation time, for paying a great deal of money to travel to Africa for this purpose, and for being willing to allow these experiences to potentially change their lives in dramatic and often disturbing ways. But even with the sincerest intentions, these people still have to "come in right." Unfortunately, many of them don't.

The first damaging story I heard in Guguletu was of an American woman who stood up at a community meeting and announced that she had met a couple of children in the township whose college educations she was going to sponsor. Of course the community cheered her announcement and thanked the woman, who then returned to the United States. The community, thinking the American would honor her commitment, assumed when there was no money forthcoming for the children's educations, that the officials in Guguletu had absconded with the money. They hadn't.

Once the American returned home, she was never heard from again. Telephone messages and e-mails to her went unanswered. It cost the community plenty for this American to visit. Young people whose hopes had been raised were disappointed. The officials who were wrongly accused of financial impropriety had their reputations damaged.

This woman didn't intentionally mislead the community. My guess is that she was overwhelmed by what she had seen and experienced, and in a moment of compassion announced something that she was simply incapable of following through on. She wasn't a bad person. It just would have been better for her to "come in right" or not come in at all.

Other visitors to the townships didn't do as much damage as this one woman, but they didn't always think before opening their mouths. At home, with our friends and families and at our jobs, most of us think twice before saying something that could be taken the wrong way or that might hurt someone's feelings. We have the ability to edit ourselves and phrase questions and comments in an appropriate manner. For some travelers, this skill seems to get lost somewhere over the Atlantic on the long flight to South Africa. Perhaps it gets left behind on the airplane with the in-flight magazine. Oh, how I wish that the lead flight attendant would make a special landing announcement to well-meaning groups of people arriving to do relief work. The message we all need to hear is:

Welcome to Cape Town, South Africa. Please remain seated with your seat belts secured until you have really listened to the following advice.

For those of you traveling to South Africa for the first time to see the townships, to learn about the history and culture of this country and the legacy of apartheid, and to meet with people living in poverty and dealing with issues such as HIV/AIDS, crime, unemployment, and lack of access to education, health care, and clean water, thank you for coming and sharing your humanity.

More than carry-on luggage and other objects may have shifted during the flight. You may feel tired, disoriented, and confused. Please take a moment to look around and make sure you have your wits about you. Remember that you are a guest in this country. You are here to listen, to learn, and to possibly respond to the issues facing this nation if you feel so moved. You are not here to judge or to intentionally or uninten-

tionally insult or disparage people whose lives you may never completely understand or identify with. You are not here to "fix" anything. Please do not attempt to put what you will see and experience into an American context. You are no longer in the United States, and viewing Africa through that lens will frustrate you and may insult your hosts, the people of South Africa. You are encouraged to ask questions and engage in active, meaningful dialogue with the people you meet. That is one way—though not the only way—to learn about life in the townships. For those of you who like to talk and ask a lot of questions, we ask that you occasionally shut up and listen. For those of you who say little but may have valuable contributions to make to discussions, we encourage you to speak up. At all times, be respectful of our people, cultures, and ways of life.

Again, welcome to South Africa. We hope you enjoy your stay and that you come in right.

That is part of the message that all of us do-gooders who travel to other parts of the world need to hear. What I have found, however, is that we do-gooders think we know all of this. We think we are different from tourists who are just on vacation. We know we are sensitive, well-intentioned people who want to make a difference in the world. We know our hearts are in the right place. We know we aren't "ugly Americans." And so, knowing all of this, we open our mouths, and sometimes ugly comments and disrespectful behavior are the result.

One man, having spent all of a few days in the townships, asked the following question based on his breadth of knowledge of South Africa: "Why is it that black women do all the work and all black men do is drink beer?"

A white woman, after keeping three people waiting for more than an hour for a scheduled meeting, walked into the meeting laughing and said, "I guess I'm just on African time."

An American minister suggested that some people with HIV/AIDS were more deserving of our support than others who had contracted the disease through "promiscuous sex." It seemed to her that there was an HIV/AIDS compassion hierarchy, with "innocent" children and "victimized" women at the top of the pyramid (those being the ones most deserving of our support) and drug-using, alcohol-abusing, sex-addicted men at the bottom (those being less worthy of our support). Therein was the lesson for that day.

Then there are those visitors who can only put what they see and experience into an American context. It's easy to see how this happens. For many, their own culture is their only frame of reference. They have left the comfort and security of their lives in the United States. One day, they are in Minneapolis, Atlanta, or New York, and a day or two later they are in Guguletu, South Africa, and suddenly things no longer make sense. They have left a black-and-white world and arrived in one made up of shades of gray. They are unstable in their new surroundings, and in reaching for some stability, they grasp on to how things operate in the West and how they as individuals operate within that world. Unfortunately, much of middle-class life in U.S. cities does not translate to a township like Guguletu.

Waiting to meet with a representative of the South African government one day, I listened to a number of American academicians in the reception area who were talking about implementing an American model to address prostitution in the townships, and thereby reduce HIV infection rates. The American model would stress self-esteem and empowerment for these women.

"What about women who don't identify as prostitutes, but who engage in transactional sex for survival?" I asked. "What about women who trade sex for food, or to pay for their children's school fees, or to just have a roof over their head that evening? Does your program offer jobs training, skills building, or education that could provide women with an alternative to survival sex or prostitution?" Although I'm simplifying their response, the answer was basically that this program had been shown to work in the United States and could be replicated in South Africa.

How did they know that? Had they met with prostitutes and women and girls engaged in survival sex? Had they listened to them in forums where the women and girls themselves had identified self-esteem as their greatest issue? Did it ever occur to them that it's not just women and girls who are engaging in these activities? That South Africa has rent boys doing the same thing? More important, did these American academicians not think that South African social issues should have South African solutions, and maybe that our role as outsiders should be to assist with those efforts instead of exporting social intervention models from the United States?

I don't claim to know the right way to come into South Africa or into any country that is new to us. I'm certain it's different for everyone. But having struggled with my own "coming in" and having accompanied scores of Americans experiencing townships for the first time, I offer this advice:

♦ *Listen more than you speak.*
♦ *Ask more than you tell.*
♦ *Behave like a guest in your boss's home.*
♦ *Resist the temptation to fix things; you might not have the tools to do so, and the thing might not be broken in the first place.*
♦ *Cast off your American lens and look at the world through different eyes.*
♦ *Don't look for simple answers for complex problems.*
♦ *Don't implement complex solutions for simple problems.*
♦ *Live with your experiences.*
♦ *If moved to act, ask what is needed. Don't assume you know.*
♦ *Be willing to make a leap of faith.*

It all boils down to what the Black Panther told Charlayne Hunter-Gault in the 1960s: "You've got to come in right."

CONTEXT

◆───

I love to travel. Sitting on a plane, returning home from a holiday, I will contemplate the next trip I want to make. If there isn't an e-ticket on my desk at all times for a trip somewhere—even a weekend getaway—I feel uneasy. My list of places to see before I die grows longer with every new stamp in my passport.

Before my work with HIV/AIDS, some of the destinations on that list included Amsterdam, Buenos Aires, and Vancouver, as well as India, Thailand, and Vietnam. Eventually, I hoped to get to Egypt and Morocco, but for the most part, the African continent held little interest for me, and I had no desire to go to South Africa. That seems odd now as I flip through a passport recording visits to Kenya, Rwanda, Uganda, and so many trips to South Africa that it necessitated having additional pages stitched into the center of my passport. Thinking back, I really don't know why South Africa was never on my radar screen to visit, though I'm sure apartheid had something to do with it.

I would like to be able to say that during my college days in the 1970s and early '80s—when Nelson Mandela was incarcerated on Robben Island—I was reading all

I could about the political situation in South Africa. In retrospect, I wish I had boycotted products of companies doing business with South Africa and that I had protested in favor of my college's divestiture of its South African investments. Today, I'm not convinced that those were necessarily the most effective methods to put pressure on the South African government to change its policies, but the effort would have counted for something. I would have done something at a time when millions of people in South Africa needed our help.

Instead, I went to college, juggling my class schedule so that it wouldn't conflict with watching *All My Children* during lunch. I worked. I went to movies, plays, concerts, restaurants, and bars. What I knew about the political situation in South Africa at the time came from one song, "Biko," that Peter Gabriel released on an album in 1980.

Stephen Biko was a young leader of South Africa's Black Consciousness movement who was beaten to death by South African police in 1977. By the time Gabriel's song was released, Mr. Biko was already a martyr of the black resistance movement. I graduated from college in 1982 with a bachelor's degree in—believe it or not—political science, without knowing anything about South African politics, except what I learned from a pop song. Had Gabriel's song not had a mesmerizing sound, I probably wouldn't have known even that much.

The South African government's policy that resulted in boycotts, demonstrations, and the deaths of people like Stephen Biko and many others was, of course, apartheid. Apartheid comes from the Afrikaans word that means "apartness." This was the white government's official pol-

icy to separate the races in South Africa. How this played
out in daily life was through laws such as:

♦ *The Prohibition of Mixed Marriages Act of 1949,
    forbidding marriage between whites and other races.*
♦ *The Population Registration Act of 1950, which
    created a national registration of everyone's race. If
    someone's race was in dispute, a Race Classification
    Board would make a determination.*
♦ *The Group Areas Act of 1950, which set aside differ-
    ent geographic areas for different races to live.*
♦ *The Suppression of Communism Act of 1950, which
    defined political activity so broadly that anyone
    demanding change could be labeled a communist
    and restricted to a specific area.*
♦ *The Prevention of Illegal Squatting Act of 1951,
    which allowed for blacks to be removed from public
    or private lands and resettled elsewhere.*
♦ *The Natives Act of 1952. Better known as Pass Laws,
    this statute required blacks to carry, at all times,
    an official identification card that included a photo-
    graph along with information on place of origin,
    tax payments, employment, and police encounters.
    It was a crime not to be in possession of one's pass
    when asked for it by the police.*
♦ *The Bantu Education Act of 1953, which created an
    official curriculum to fit the "nature and require-
    ments of the black people."*
♦ *The Reservation of Separate Amenities Act of 1953,
    which authorized separate and unequal public
    amenities for anyone who wasn't white. "European*

*Only" and "Non-Europeans Only" signs began to
be used to further separate the races.*
♦ *The Terrorism Act of 1967, which allowed the government to detain, indefinitely, prisoners without
trial.*

One of the many aspects of apartheid that I will never
understand is that the policies started to be implemented
by South Africa's National Party just a few years after the
end of World War II. At a time when the entire world
had to confront the Holocaust and the lack of international outrage over those atrocities as they were occurring, South Africa enacted laws based on the alleged
superiority of whites. And, for the most part, the world
looked the other way.

In part because of laws like the Group Areas Act, the
township system began to develop in South Africa. The
races were separated, and nonwhites, including blacks, col-
oureds (persons of mixed-race background), and Indians,
were relocated to different areas adjoining "whites-only"
communities so as to provide white residents and businesses with a cheap and plentiful work force.

Johannesburg has townships such as Soweto (which
stands for South West Townships), and Cape Town has
townships like Khayelitsha and Guguletu. More recently,
in the post-apartheid era, thousands of people are flocking
to urban townships from rural areas in search of opportunities and better lives. Seemingly overnight, squatter
camps appear—houses made from whatever scrounged
materials its inhabitants can find. These informal settle-

ments often lack water and access to electricity. There's no heat source for the cold, damp winters. If a fire breaks out it quickly spreads from shack to shack before it can be extinguished, often leaving people injured or dead and hundreds of others homeless.

Now, I'm not a historian or a sociologist or a medical doctor. I don't claim to be an expert on South Africa, poverty, or even on HIV/AIDS. However, I strongly believe that one cannot begin to understand the HIV/AIDS epidemic in South Africa without some context concerning the historical, political, and social events that, decade after decade, helped create an environment that was ripe for the eventual spread of a catastrophic public health crisis like HIV/AIDS.

It's not enough, as some Americans have said to me, to suggest that HIV/AIDS has spread in Africa and other parts of the developing world because "those people" have a different sense of morality. We must put this health crisis—and others—into context. One is incapable of comprehending HIV/AIDS in South Africa without also learning something about the country's history and the role of apartheid in that history.

I wish I had paid more attention when some of the history I now read about was occurring. I wish I had been more involved with the issue of apartheid when it was critical that people made their opinions known and their voices heard. There is nothing I can do now about my lack of interest and involvement during the antiapartheid movement of the 1970s and '80s, but there is something I can do about the issue of today: HIV/AIDS.

In the 1980s I listened to Peter Gabriel's song about Stephen Biko and heard the remarkable words "and the eyes of the world are watching now." At the time I thought it was little more than a catchy tagline to a great song. I see now that it was a call to action.

PAUL THEROUX IS SMARTER THAN I AM

◆───────────────────────────────

The writer Paul Theroux is much smarter than I am. He's more talented, and he is certainly better traveled than I am. In his book *Dark Star Safari,* Theroux chronicles his travels from Cairo, Egypt, to Cape Town, South Africa. Only a select few, including Nobel laureate Nadine Gordimer and some "bare-assed" Africans he met along his journey, escape Theroux's cynical and pessimistic comments. Some of his harshest criticisms are reserved for international aid experts and charity workers, who, according to Theroux, range from "selfless idealists" to the "laziest boondogglers." On the Theroux spectrum of Western interlopers, I suspect I would be labeled an idealistic charity worker, though not entirely selfless. "Charities and aid programs," Theroux writes, "seemed to turn African problems into permanent conditions that were bigger and messier."

OK, Mr. Theroux may be right. He is not the only person who thinks international aid is nothing more than handouts that deprive Africans of their dignity and ambition. And, as I said, this acclaimed author is smarter than I am and has experienced more of the African continent than I have. But, of all the places Theroux describes in his book, there is one that I feel confident in saying that I know better: Guguletu.

Theroux devotes a couple of pages in the second-to-last chapter of his 472-page book to Guguletu. He mentions Amy Biehl, the American Fulbright scholar who was brutally murdered in Guguletu. He describes the handmade sign posted near the memorial site of her killing as "so crude as to be insulting." He calls the argument that Biehl's murderers made before the Truth and Reconciliation Commission as "ridiculous," "lame," and "without merit." He writes about the shacks and shops and shebeens of the township. He mentions the circumcision school that he noticed off the highway in Guguletu.

My experiences in Guguletu are different from Mr. Theroux's.

The Biehl memorial is near the Caltex gas station where I fill up my tank and talk to its owner. The handwritten sign in memory of Amy is crude, but it is not insulting. I, too, have spent time in countless township shacks, shops, and shebeens, and I didn't just drive by the circumcision camp along the highway. Along with my host, I spent an afternoon at circumcision school meeting with young Xhosa men who had just gone through the long-standing ritual and shared ginger beer with them in their smoke-filled huts.

Before transitioning from the morning he spent in Guguletu to his stay at a "magnificent country house hotel, the Grande Roche Luxury Estate Hotel," later that same day, Theroux describes the inhabitants of Guguletu and a neighboring squatter camp called New Rest as being "so grateful, all they wished for was to make their shacks more permanent, so they could stay there for the rest of their lives."

In Theroux's entire book, nothing stood out to me as more inaccurate—as just plain wrong—as this single sentence. But, Theroux is smarter than I am, and much more talented and better traveled, so who was I to question him?

So I didn't question him. Instead, I questioned people who live in Guguletu and the surrounding squatter camps. I asked them a simple question: "What is it that you wish for?"

None of them expressed a wish to "make their shacks more permanent." That is not to say that housing wasn't at the top of some people's wish list, but if they lived in a shack in a squatter's camp, their wish wasn't to make it more permanent—it was to move out.

Bongiwe is twenty years old and a member of a singing group in Guguletu called Siyaya. When the group gets performance gigs, they are usually late at night, and it's not uncommon for Bongiwe to be returning to the shack she stays in with her family at 1:00 in the morning or later.

"Sometimes when I come back late from a performance," Bongiwe told me, "I'm scared that someone will attack me while I wait for my mom to open the door. It's not a safe place for my family to live. I wish that one day I could have a house for my family, not a shack, away from the crime."

Nomsa had thought about her dreams long before I asked her what she wished for. Without a second's hesitation, she said: "OK, my first wish is that I would like my father to go to church. Secondly, if there was a magic wand, I would wish for all the people dying of AIDS to be healthy. My third wish is that I would have my own house. I like writing poetry, and I need time for myself to be on my own. And my fourth wish is for my younger brother to be happy."

Mr. Theroux's observation that all people want is to make their shacks more permanent, certainly does not apply to Nomsa. She really wants a place of her own. She really needs a place of her own. A year before I met Nomsa she had swallowed thirty sleeping tablets in a suicide attempt. A neighbor found her unconscious and got her to a hospital. Nomsa gets counseling now and she is doing better, but sometimes the stress of her living situation, all of those people in such a small space, gets to be too much for her.

I asked sixteen people what they wished for and yes, a few wished for a big house and a nice car. One wished for a swimming pool. Many wished for clothes, new clothes, warm clothes, fancy clothes. Some wished to be successful. Thobile wished that I could put him in my suitcase and take him to America.

Silas also wanted to come to the United States, but his motivation was different from Thobile's. "I want to meet some other people and gain some experience about other people. I want to ask them why they don't have HIV. What's their secret why they don't have HIV like we do? I want to please ask them for the recipe to not get HIV. Maybe there is something different about them physically or mentally. There are many things I want to know in life."

I was driving to Carnation Hospital one day with Gloria and Baba when I asked them what they wished for. Gloria has AIDS, and although she has nearly died on occasion, she retains her tremendous spirit. Perhaps what keeps Gloria going is her single wish: to live for another four years so that she can see her sixteen-year-old son go to circumcision school, where, in Xhosa culture, he will become a man. Once he has been to the "bush," as circumcision schools are called, then Gloria's son can take care of himself, and she will no longer need to worry about him.

Baba, who is also HIV-positive, has a huge personality that cannot be contained in the compact car we're driving in. I tell her that when she is with me I have to drive with the windows open to release some of the energy that builds up in the car when she talks. When we talk about wishes, however, Baba becomes very quiet.

"I just wish to live longer," was her reply to my question—the most concise response I got from anyone I talked with about their wishes.

Nolusindiso is thirty-one. She prefers to be called Cindy. Ever since her father died two years ago, her family has been in turmoil. She shares her mother's house with ten other family members. As many as possible fit into the two beds in the house, and the rest sleep on pieces of foam rubber on the floor. The family's main problem is not enough food. Some days, there is nothing to eat, not even rice. The family goes to bed at night having eaten nothing all day.

"It's hard to watch the kids go to school because there isn't even money for bread to take with them. This thing is getting to my mother. She is very much stressed as she watches what is happening to us. We are becoming a joke within the community. But they don't know that we go to bed with no food. Our kids don't have school uniforms, so it's evident that we are very poor. What's painful is that winter is coming and our kids don't have any clothing for winter. Since it's been two years since my father died, that's the last time they had clothes and now they have outgrown them. The only prayer I have within me is that I can make life more bearable at my house. Stress has taken me to the far ends."

And what does Cindy wish for?

"First, I would buy groceries for the family. It has always bothered me that our kids go to school with nothing to eat. Maybe with food, they could concentrate and do well at school. I would buy shoes for my daughter and my sister so they have shoes for the winter. Maybe I could buy them uniforms so they don't look different than other children at school. I think if I could make some money, my mother would get some relief and maybe be happy for once. I don't feature in my wishes. First, it's the children and my mother. Then we must fix the house to stop the leaks in the roof."

Linda's wish is uniquely his. Two years ago he was in a car accident that resulted in his face being disfigured. Linda lives for music, for singing. It is all he knows how to

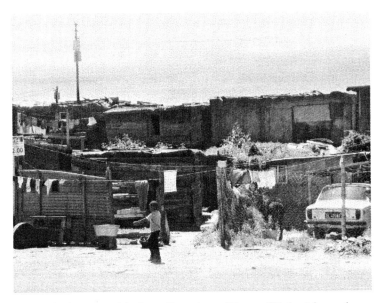

Paul Theroux said about Guguletu: "It was filled with people so grateful, all they wished for was to make their shacks more permanent, so they could stay there for the rest of their lives." The people I know in Guguletu wish for much more.

do, and it's all he wants to do for a career. He is starting to get paid for performing at restaurants and tourist venues, but he told me: "I see when I perform how people look at me. When something is wrong with your face, it's like people are judging you. I wish to have a doctor to mend my face. I just hope people see me as a person, not a scar."

As Linda was walking out of the room where we had been talking, he added: "There's still glass in my face and it hurts. If a doctor could fix my face, maybe he could get the glass out."

I understand that Paul Theroux lives in Hawaii. I have no idea what he wishes for, but I'm guessing it's not renovating his home so that he can stay there forever.

I have a laundry list of wishes and most of them are self-centered. I have added another wish to my list, however, and this one is a bit more altruistic. I wish that Paul Theroux would spend more time in Guguletu and that in subsequent reprintings of *Dark Star Safari,* he would revise the sentence that says that all people wish for is to make their shacks more permanent and to live there for the rest of their lives.

HOW COULD WE HAVE LET THIS HAPPEN?

◆————————————————————————————

In *A Problem from Hell,* Pulitzer Prize–winning writer Samantha Power discusses genocide and describes how the United States failed to respond to the mass exterminations of people in Cambodia, Iraq, Bosnia, and Rwanda. In case after case, our government—and eventually all of us—knew what was happening in those countries. Only after the killings stopped did we wring our hands and say, "How could we have let this happen?"

I have been in South Africa less than one month and I have already lost track of the number of times I have asked myself this same question about HIV/AIDS: "How can we be letting this happen?"

In KwaZulu-Natal, the northern province of South Africa, there is a nonprofit organization providing care to people living with HIV/AIDS called Amangwe Village. They have their hands full. KwaZulu-Natal has the highest HIV prevalence rate in all of South Africa.

As part of their program, Amangwe supports a sixteen-bed hospital. When I visited, all the beds were full. Fifteen of the sixteen patients had HIV/AIDS. Before patients can be admitted, they must inform the hospital which funeral home is in charge of their arrangements should they die at Amangwe. An energetic and dedicated social worker gave me a tour of the hospital. As we neared the end of the tour (it didn't take long, there is only a male ward and a female ward), my host casually pointed out the "corpse room" where bodies are kept until family members come to claim them. As I drove away from Amangwe Village, I passed a local cemetery. The scores of fresh graves confirmed the toll HIV/AIDS is taking on this community.

◆

At the opposite end of the country, an HIV/AIDS support group meets every Tuesday evening in Guguletu, South Africa. The Zwane Community Centre provides hot soup on a bitingly cold winter's night to the participants. I'm introduced to a young woman bundled in a heavy coat, knit cap, and gloves. She had two children, both of them born HIV-positive. On the day of her daughter's funeral, the mother arrived home to find that her only surviving child, her son, had died that afternoon as she was burying her daughter.

Another day at the community center in Guguletu, I hear a woman call my name. She teaches in the after-school program, and I had met her on a visit to South Africa the previous year. She greets me and says, "Remember my cousin and niece? They're both gone now. AIDS."

As I'm leaving the center one night, I run into Zethu Xapile, the nurse who runs Brown's Farm Clinic and also leads the HIV/AIDS support group. As she talks about her day she tells me that she tested nine people for HIV—five of them were positive. "It's always about fifty percent positive," she tells me. The pain on her face betrays her matter-of-fact recitation of the statistics.

In Cape Town, I catch a cab to take me home from the waterfront one evening. The cab driver tells me he lives in the Cape Flats. I ask him where in the Flats he lives, and when he tells me "Khayelitsha," he is surprised that I have been there.

"Why do you go to Khayelitsha?" he asks. By mentioning HIV/AIDS, I give him permission to talk. And talk he does—all the way to my apartment where he turns off the cab and continues to talk.

"My wife has 'H.' I don't have 'H' " (an even more concise abbreviation for HIV, which I have heard several times since arriving in South Africa). "Every night I rub my wife's feet and her legs and her hands because they are numb. I don't mind. I love her. Please, can I ask you something? How do I get her those pills?"

I tell the taxi driver about the project in Khayelitsha, where Doctors Without Borders is providing free antiretroviral medications to about 500 people. What I don't tell him is that hundreds of thousands of people in South Africa are in situations similar to his wife's—waiting to somehow get the drugs they hope will save their lives.

At some point in our future, someone will write a book that details how tens of millions of people died of HIV/AIDS as governments debated policies, the media concentrated on other issues, donors funded other priorities, and individuals thought there was little they could do—if they thought about HIV/AIDS at all. And yet again, we will wring our hands and say, "How could we have let this happen?"

SOUTH AFRICA'S GREATEST IN-LINER (BY NEXT YEAR THIS TIME)

◆────────────────────────────────

I met South Africa's greatest in-line skater today. At least he will be "by next year this time."

Bheki Kunene is an energetic, confident young Xhosa man who has a comfort with his body that you don't often see in a fifteen-year-old male. For seven of his years—nearly half his life—Bheki has been rollerblading. Owning just three pairs of skates during that time, Bheki has become "one of the greatest rollerbladers in Guguletu." That's a quote from a sponsorship request I received from him while I was living in South Africa and working at the Zwane Community Centre in the township of Guguletu.

Bheki lives at NY7-46 in Guguletu. The old apartheid government didn't believe the black townships warranted names for their neighborhoods, so they gave them codes. The "NY" stands for "native yards." The poor black youth of Guguletu live in neighborhoods with names like NY7. The wealthy white youth of Cape Town live in neighborhoods with names like Constantia.

Bheki and his mom share a home with his grandmother, his auntie, and his cousin. His uncle just moved to Durban in hopes of finding a job. With unemployment at about 65 percent in Guguletu, you have to believe the uncle's move was a good one.

The self-proclaimed "greatest rollerblader of Guguletu" knows how to write a letter that will appeal to sponsors. In addition to describing his passion for the sport, Bheki informs prospective benefactors that skating "keeps me away from the streets." As cognizant as Bheki is of himself and his surroundings, the poetry of his own statement escapes him. A sport that, for the most part, exists for the street is also what allows a young black man to safely navigate through the threats and temptations of "the streets." And the streets of Guguletu are not easy.

There is only one obstacle to Bheki's dream of becoming South Africa's greatest in-line skater "by next year this time."

He doesn't have in-line skates.

Bheki tried to explain how rollerblades are different than the in-line skates one needs to do tricks and become a professional skater, but the differences were lost on me. I took him at his word when he said that he has gone as far as he can in the in-line skating world with his current blades. Besides, this isn't a story about skating. This is a story about dreams.

Haven't we all wanted something in life so badly that we actually dreamt about it? I did. When I was younger than Bheki is now, I wanted a guitar so much that I could think of nothing else. One Christmas, after everyone else had opened their presents, out came a black case with a brand-new guitar in it for me. I knew that my parents had saved long and hard to buy that guitar. They must have been disappointed when, after a particularly painful lesson,

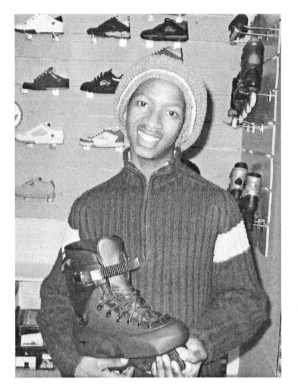

*Sometimes, the most important thing you can do
is buy a kid a pair of skates.*

the guitar never came out of its case again. But even though
I abandoned the guitar, my parents had given me a much
more important gift. I knew from a young age that dreams
really could come true.

Who will make Bheki's dreams come true?

Bheki's mom tried. It's universal—mothers always
try. Bheki saved money by taking the train to school instead of the bus. His mother chipped in what she could.

Altogether their efforts yielded enough rand for Bheki to buy a helmet, which was mandatory if he was going to practice at skating parks. Bheki says mathematics is his favorite subject in school. He did the math. He could take the train to school for a year and still would not have saved enough money for in-line skates.

It may seem indulgent to think about helping one kid in a township to get a pair of expensive skates when thousands of others go hungry and thousands more dream of receiving the AIDS drugs that could prolong their lives. But I always remember one of my mother's adages: "Where there's life, there's hope." And there must be hope.

Bheki is both life and hope. He is overflowing with optimism and confidence and vitality in a neighborhood—no, in a *world*—that does not have enough of these traits.

Those of us born into the power and privilege that come with being white can never imagine the courage it took for a young black kid from the townships to make an appointment with a white guy from America to share his dream of becoming "South Africa's greatest in-liner."

The hopes and dreams those in-line skates represent—*they* are worth investing in. For Bheki . . . and for us.

LUNDI'S STORY

♦

It was Lundi Ntikinca whose body was laid out before
me at the Trinity International Funeral Supply Company,
but I was the one having an out-of-body experience.

Lundi's family, his teenage daughter, an aunt, some
cousins, his girlfriend, and I all gathered around the metal
examination table that supported Lundi's body in a small
visitation room at the funeral supply company. The walls
were painted the color of split-pea soup, and the green
wall behind me displayed expensive metal handles and
trimmings in gold and silver should a bereaved family
want to upgrade their loved one's casket. A floor lamp in
the corner illuminated Lundi's head, the only part of his
body not covered by a threadbare white sheet dotted with
pastel blue diamonds.

It seemed odd—impossible, really—that a corpse could
look good in this poorly lit, garishly painted room, but
Lundi did look good. He looked much better than the last
time I saw him, three weeks earlier at an HIV/AIDS support group. His face had been shaved, and Lundi's tight
braids pillowed his head on the metal table. I had been
surprised to learn that Lundi was only thirty-four years old
when he died. He looked much older. But today, stand-

ing with the family looking down at his body, I thought Lundi looked younger and more handsome.

The elderly aunt with whom Lundi lived began to pray in Xhosa. Lundi's daughter and girlfriend stood crying while his cousins and best friend took a few steps back from the body. Lundi's aunt had to compete to be heard with the sounds of drilling and sawing coming from the warehouse that was just behind the thin wall of the reviewal room. Someone in the warehouse turned up the volume on the radio, and the sound of Phil Collins singing "True Colors" filled the room and drowned out the aunt's voice. The cousins and best friend moved closer to hear what she was saying.

I was transfixed. I had been invited by the family to participate in the planning of Lundi's funeral, but the background noise, the color of the room, Lundi's body, and the solemn events that were unfolding before me caused me to disconnect with the moment. I realized that although I was in the room, I was really only an observer. It was as though I were a medical student watching a surgery from an observatory above the operating room.

I was jarred from my trance by the obnoxious buzzing of the funeral director's cell phone. I was even more startled when the funeral director, who was standing next to me, began to talk on the phone while the grieving family stood only a few feet away from her. Now, in addition to the music and the drilling and sawing, the prayers had to compete with a phone conversation.

When the family stopped praying, the funeral director took that as her cue to say a quick "Ciao" and put the phone in her purse. She then walked up to the corpse, addressed him by name, and said a few sentences in Xhosa before covering Lundi's head with the sheet and motioning for us to leave the room. Outside, another family stood by the coffins, waiting for their turn to view a body.

Later that night, alone in my apartment, I replayed the day's events. When I closed my eyes I saw Lundi's dead face, the green walls, and the white-and-blue sheet. If I think about it now, years later, I can still see that scene. Something in my head, or my heart, shut off that day to allow me to do what needed to be done. But that momentary out-of-body experience in the viewing room left a lasting image in my mind. It's an image I can't delete like I could an unwanted snapshot taken with a digital camera. Lundi's dead face, the green walls, and the white-and-blue sheet: they are what I see whenever I begin to tell Lundi's story.

I only remember speaking to Lundi once. He was a member of an HIV/AIDS support group in Guguletu that I regularly attended to get a better understanding of the pandemic in South Africa. In recognition of World AIDS Day, the group had decided to write their personal stories about living with HIV/AIDS. They asked me to take photos of members so that they could include pictures in their World AIDS Day exhibit. I would snap a photo and then show the person their image on the screen of the digital camera. The expressions on their faces when they saw themselves confirmed that many members of the group had never seen a digital camera before.

As I was taking pictures of other support group members, I noticed Lundi sitting straight in his chair, pointing at himself—a clear indication that he wanted his photo taken. I liked the photo that appeared in the screen after I pushed the shoot button of my camera. Lundi was like many other people in the township who want their photos taken, but won't look directly into the lens. The image that appeared showed Lundi looking slightly away from the camera. What I liked about it was that he had just the slightest hint of a smile on his face. Many times the same people who don't want to look at a camera also don't want to smile for their picture, but when I showed Lundi his image in the screen, he said "OK" and I moved on to the next person.

Ten minutes later, I was still taking pictures when Lundi came up to me and asked to see his image again. I scrolled through dozens of photos on my digital camera until Lundi's face reappeared. Lundi looked at it for a moment and said, "No. Another photo." I was curious as to what it was about this one that Lundi didn't like. "It's bad. I have a smile." Lundi sat down in the same chair and I took a second photo of him still looking away from the camera, but this time a serious expression replaced the smile. The following week I brought copies of the photos to the support group and distributed them to everyone there. It was the last time I saw Lundi until I was standing above his corpse at the funeral supply company.

♦

Lundi had been dead for two days before I learned of his death. An acquaintance, Mandla Majola of South Africa's powerful AIDS activist group, the Treatment Action Campaign (TAC), had left a message on my cell phone. Using the language of TAC, Mandla informed me that a "comrade" in the fight against AIDS had died, and his death had created an "especially difficult situation." Would I meet with Mandla to discuss the situation?

I assumed that the "difficult situation" was that there was no money to pay for Lundi's funeral. Even before AIDS, life in townships like Guguletu was difficult. With 65 percent unemployment and a historically inadequate educational system, it's nearly impossible for families to work their way out of poverty. AIDS has destroyed many families because it is young people such as Lundi—the very ones who should be working and supporting their extended families—who are getting sick and dying, leaving elderly relatives to care for surviving children and pay for funerals. Before calling Mandla back, I checked to see how much money I had to contribute to a funeral, should that be what he was calling about.

Mandla was tired and sick the next morning when we met in Guguletu. He had a weariness about him that would not disappear with rest. Years of involvement in the struggle against apartheid and now HIV/AIDS appeared to have taken a toll on him. As I drank coffee and Mandla swallowed aspirin, the "difficult situation" began to unfold. It was a difficult situation, but not an uncommon one.

Lundi hadn't been able to work for a long time; consequently, he had no money saved and hadn't contributed to any of the popular funeral savings plans that are widely promoted around South Africa. Lundi's parents were dead. He lived with an aunt and uncle who supported the entire extended family on the aunt's old-age pension of less than 600 rand (approximately $100 a month). I didn't ask about the mother of Lundi's four children or what would happen to the children now that their father had died. Families in South Africa try their best to care for orphans, and I assumed the same would be true for Lundi's children. The immediate problem was that there was no money to pay for a funeral. If the money could not be found, eventually the government would claim Lundi's body at the funeral supply company and bury it in an undisclosed location. Mandla turned to me and said, "I can't let that happen to a comrade and a friend."

Mandla would ask TAC to provide buses for transporting the mourners to and from the cemetery. Lundi's church would provide sandwiches and refreshments for lunch following the funeral. The greatest expense, the actual cost of the funeral, was what I was being asked to underwrite. Friends in the United States had given me money to assist in cases like this, but even if I didn't have that resource, I still would have assisted with this difficult situation—not so much because of Lundi, whom I really didn't know—but because of Mandla's impassioned appeal on behalf of his dead friend. I was about to offer my assistance when Mandla said there was one more component to this request. Would I also meet with the family and help them make the funeral arrangements?

The minister of Lundi's church, who had also been sitting in on this meeting, finally joined the conversation. He said it would be good for me to see firsthand how the death of a person from AIDS affects a family in South Africa. "If you really want to understand the AIDS pandemic at a human level," he said, "this is the way to do it."

Sometimes it's best not to think too long before making a decision. I had no way of knowing where this experience would take me, but I immediately said yes to assisting with the funeral costs and to working with a family I had never met. Thirty minutes later, I was sitting in Lundi's home being introduced to his family.

Except for the aunt's worn rocking chair, the furniture in the living room had already been removed from the room, replaced with roughhewn wooden benches for mourners to sit on. From the time a person dies until the funeral—which can sometimes be weeks—mourners call on the family every night for prayers. Usually, the family is expected to provide food and drink to anyone who calls; but in Lundi's case, there was no money, and consequently there were no refreshments to offer visitors.

Sitting on benches, with Mandla interpreting in Xhosa, I explained to the family that I would pay for the most basic and inexpensive funeral we could arrange. It was an awkward meeting. I was there to talk about death and money. The family didn't know me, yet they needed my assistance. Often we would all sit in silence. Eventually, it was agreed that I would return to their home the following Monday to meet with the funeral director to plan the funeral and discuss actual costs.

Before leaving, I remembered that I had brought copies of the two photos I had taken of Lundi—the one with a hint of a smile and the one with the serious expression that Lundi liked. I showed them to the aunt, who passed them to the others sitting on the benches that lined the walls. Lundi's cousin asked if I would make copies of the photos so that they could be used for the funeral. It was a unanimous decision on which photo to use—the one with the serious expression. Lundi would have been pleased.

◆

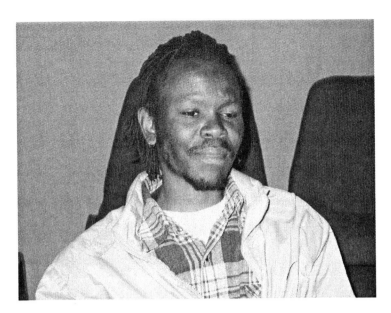

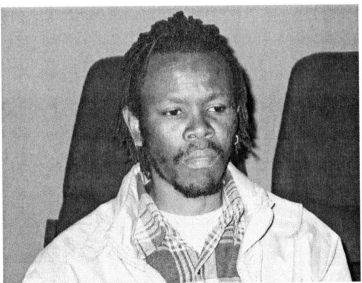

Lundi just weeks before he died. I preferred the photo with the slight smile. Lundi preferred the serious one.

Lundi had now been dead nearly a week when I returned to his aunt's house with copies of Lundi's photograph, to meet again with the family and also with the funeral director. On this, my second visit, the family seemed a bit more relaxed. I was a bit more anxious. I know how funerals are arranged in the States, but I had no idea what happens in the townships of South Africa. There also was the matter of money that needed to be finalized. I had been told the previous week that a basic funeral would cost about six hundred dollars. I was determined not to exceed that amount, because any money I gave toward a funeral would be money that could not go to support the needs of someone living. Still, I know the role emotion plays in situations like these, so I steeled myself against the possibility that the family or the funeral director might ask for more than I was willing to pay.

After the preliminary handshakes and greetings, we all sat down again on the same wooden benches that were still in place for the evening mourners. And, like the previous meeting, there were periods of silence between exchanges. Eventually, I turned to Mandla from TAC and asked what we were waiting for. I assumed that we would be going to a funeral home, but Mandla explained that the funeral director, Nomfundo Mlamla, would actually come to the house to discuss the arrangements. While we waited, Lundi's cousin took one of the photos of Lundi that I had brought with me and taped it high on a wall above the chair where Lundi's aunt was sitting.

When the funeral director arrived, the silence was shattered. Nomfundo greeted each family member and immediately got down to business. Mandla explained who

I was and that I was contributing toward the costs of the funeral, but that didn't mean that this was going to be an expensive funeral. Mandla was there to ensure that I wasn't overcharged.

Item by item, Nomfundo recited the costs with Mandla taking notes. "Forty dollars to remove the body from the hospital. Fifty-seven dollars to store the body until burial. Fifty dollars for the hearse. One hundred and forty-five dollars for the coffin . . ." Would I pay for buses to transport the mourners to the cemetery? "No." TAC had said they would consider paying that cost, and I wanted to make sure others contributed to the funeral. What about food for the lunch afterward? Would I assist with those costs? "No." Again, the church said it would ask members and neighbors to provide the food. It was important to me that the community had some role in Lundi's funeral, even if it was only to provide sandwiches.

The details of the funeral decided, everyone stood up and began putting on jackets and walking out the front door of the aunt's small house. The aunt, a large woman, used her cane to lift herself from her chair, and a grandchild brought her coat and hat. I assumed our meeting was finished and that I would return to work when Mandla said that the family was now going to the funeral home to pick out the casket, and it was assumed that I would accompany them to the Trinity Funeral Supply Company.

Trinity Funeral Supply Company. The very name suggests a no-frills operation, and Trinity Funeral Supply Company is the Sam's Club of the funeral business—only not as upscale as Sam's Club. This wasn't a funeral home like in the West, and it certainly wasn't a funeral parlor.

There was no soft music playing, no green plants in a large, carpeted lobby. There were no comfortable chairs to sit on with tissue boxes strategically placed on end tables. There were no pleasant employees to meet us at the door, shake our hands, and convey their condolences.

A couple of folding chairs were against the wall. Lundi's aunt, girlfriend, and daughter sat, while the rest of us stood on the worn, soiled carpet. Two employees sat at a dirty receptionist desk, smoking cigarettes. They stopped their conversation long enough to look at us when we entered, and then resumed speaking to one another, never bothering to say hello as they blew smoke in our direction.

Nomfundo, the funeral director who had come to Lundi's house to meet with us, was nowhere to be seen. I discovered later that she was in the warehouse from which the sound of sawing, drilling, and Phil Collins music was emanating, checking on the status of Lundi's body. When she appeared a few minutes later, she showed us around the corner into a small U-shaped room packed with caskets from which we could select one.

Cheap wooden caskets were placed next to the more expensive metal ones. A shiny metallic blue coffin with faux-silk lining was the focal point of the room. It was by far the most expensive casket and hands down the most hideous. Plastic flowers wrapped in cellophane or stuffed into clear plastic bags were hanging on the walls and were scattered randomly on the coffins. No effort was made to properly display any of the merchandise, and no attempt was made to somehow soften what we were here to do. This really was a funeral supply company. If you wanted a funeral parlor, you needed to go elsewhere, where you would pay accordingly for the service.

"This is the box you want," Nomfundo said as Lundi's family and I were looking at other caskets in the room. "It's the cheapest one we have."

We turned to face the funeral director, and her assertion was correct. Lundi would not be buried in a plush casket. He would be laid to rest in a box. From a distance, it didn't look bad. The pressed wood had been painted white and the edges trimmed in black brush strokes to suggest a box more substantial and attractive than it really was. On closer inspection, I wondered if the wood was even strong enough to hold Lundi's emaciated corpse. Nomfundo unscrewed the quarter-inch lid of the box so that we could see inside. There was no pillow and no pad for the body to rest on, just a white plastic lining that looked like a heavy-duty garbage bag that served a specific function none of us wanted to discuss.

Lundi's cousin approached me and said, "Is this all right with you? We think it's OK, if you do. The others cost too much."

"It's good. I like it," I said. And I wasn't lying. Most of the other caskets were gaudy. There was a simplicity to this one that appealed to me.

At that moment, a family came out from the tiny room that adjoined the casket showroom. A young woman was sobbing, distraught, supported by a man on either side of her who were escorting her out of the funeral supply company. It was then that I realized that we would be the next group escorted into that tiny, green-walled room to view Lundi's body for the last time before it was returned to the aunt's house for the funeral.

Lundi's funeral, like most funerals in the townships, would be on Saturday. Having funerals on Saturdays gives time for family members who have to travel from rural areas to get to Guguletu. It also means that those fortunate few people who are employed don't have to take time off from work to attend a funeral. After this one meeting at the funeral supply company, the remainder of my time with the family would be at the home of Lundi's aunt, where the funeral would take place.

Part of the funeral costs I agreed to pay was for the rental of a white-and-blue carnival-type tent that was draped from the front of Lundi's aunt's house, over the yard and to the street. Plastic sides were zipped in to create an enclosure protected from the cool winds that can blow at night in Guguletu. The tent created a large space for mourners to gather, but it also created obstacles as guests, in order to avoid tripping and falling, had to step over the steel spikes and ropes that secured the tent.

The Thursday before the funeral, I returned to the house to pay the funeral director. I carefully inspected the detailed receipt, and slowly counted out 3,900 rand (the equivalent of $600) as the family all watched. With a receipt in hand, I left to a chorus of "enkosi kakhulu," and instructions from the family to be back at the house by 9:00 a.m. on Saturday for the funeral.

A young friend once told me she hates Saturdays in Guguletu because "it's boring. Everyone is at a funeral."

It's easy to find a house in the township on the day of a funeral. You look for the tent and the crowds of people and activity. Of course, you need to make sure you are on the right street because there are a number of funerals every Saturday in the townships. Lundi's funeral was not the only one along the street this particular Saturday. His was, however, the only funeral that had the Treatment Action Campaign banner demanding access to medications stretched across the front of the tent.

Lundi's minister had informed me that this service would be as much a political event as it would be a religious funeral. This was obvious by the number of mourners who arrived wearing the uniform of TAC: white T-shirts with "HIV Positive" printed on them in large purple letters.

As the funeral was about to begin, a few visitors from the United States and I were escorted toward the front of the house. We were seated directly across from Lundi's aunt and other women mourners. The men, Lundi's cousins and friends, all stood toward the back of the tent, for the most part, away from the women.

The gathering stood as they sang in Xhosa and Lundi's casket was brought out from the house and placed on sawhorses beneath a wire arch decorated with red, orange, blue, green, and white plastic flowers and strips of ribbon. The sides of the tent had been removed to allow for a breeze on this warm spring morning. The casket came to rest directly in front of me. Two bouquets of plastic flowers that I had seen at the funeral supply company, still wrapped in cellophane, were placed on top of the casket, as were a handful of letters and cards. Lundi's yellow Treatment Action Campaign T-shirt was draped over the end of the casket.

I was so close to the coffin that whenever I stood for a prayer or a song, my body brushed against it. If I crossed my leg, my foot touched the casket. At one point during the service, when Lundi's aunt reached across the white box to give the minister a letter, I braced the sawhorses with my feet and steadied the casket with my hands, afraid the weight of Lundi's aunt could disturb the delicately balanced box and cause it to crash to the ground.

Bonga, a young volunteer from TAC, was the emcee of the funeral. In Xhosa, he introduced family members to speak and ministers to preach. The mourners knew when to sit for the singing of an AIDS protest song and when to rise for the singing of a hymn, but I found the protocol confusing. Eventually, a woman sitting behind me whispered in my ear that I should just sit for the remainder of the funeral. That would be proper, she said.

Nearing the end of the service, Lundi's cousin came from the back of the tent and asked me to follow him to the street. Outside of the tent he told me that I would shortly be expected to speak to the crowd. I told him that I preferred not to speak and would just stand with him outside of the tent for the remainder of the funeral. He nodded in what I took to be a sign of agreement. A few minutes later he said, "It's time for you to speak. You must go back inside now."

As I walked back toward my chair, Lundi's aunt began moving toward the emcee, who motioned for me to join them at the front of the house and at the head of Lundi's casket. I could hardly squeeze past the first row of mourners and Lundi's coffin to face the assembled mourners.

Speaking in English, Lundi's aunt called me her son and

said that there would have been no funeral without me. On behalf of Lundi's children and the people of Guguletu, she thanked me for helping her family. I don't remember what I said to the congregation, but I do remember thinking, even as the words were coming out of my mouth, how insipid I sounded. A minister during the funeral had said something about "standing together," and I closed my comments by saying I was happy to "stand with the people of Guguletu in their struggle against HIV/AIDS." Ugh.

The two-hour service over, I drove again to the cemetery in Guguletu, where I would spend many Saturdays during my time in South Africa, and watched that white box being lowered into the ground and covered with dirt. Then I returned with the others to Lundi's aunt's house, washed my hands in the buckets of water outside the tent, and sat down for a lunch of sandwiches prepared by neighbors and members of the church.

The day of the funeral, Lundi's aunt asked me to visit her before I returned to the United States. I still had months left of my stay in South Africa, and I think I surprised her by the number of times I visited, usually bringing groceries for her family and always suckers for her three-year-old grandson, who would exclaim "Cavin!" every time I saw him.

Lundi's aunt thought that I was visiting her for some altruistic reason, or out of some sense of obligation and responsibility. The truth is, I visited her and her family because it made me feel good. It made me feel that I could do something to make a positive difference in the lives of this one family. It made me feel that maybe something good could come from all of the misery that AIDS has caused the world; that AIDS has caused this family; that AIDS has caused me.

I have always believed that something good can come from this horrific disease.

I have to believe that.

It's the only way the world can make sense to me anymore.

A FULL-SERVICE STATION

◆————————————————————————————————

In August of 1993, Amy Biehl, an American Fulbright scholar, was murdered in Guguletu along the NY1, one of the main roads of the township. At the time, the political nature of her murder generated international media attention. The story received even more attention when Amy's parents testified before South Africa's post-apartheid Truth and Reconciliation Commission in support of the killers being released from prison. In the decade since Amy's death, the Biehls have created a foundation in their daughter's memory to address the social and economic needs of people living in townships like Guguletu. Some of the foundation's projects have, at times, employed two of the men involved with Amy's death.

A stone marker identifies the spot near the road where Amy Biehl was murdered. When friends visit from the States, I take them to the monument. Most visitors have some memory of an American who was killed in South Africa, but others have never heard of Amy Biehl. Either way, a visit to the monument provides an opportunity to talk about the young woman who lived her ideals, and how a family turned a tragedy into a legacy.

There's a Caltex gas station located directly behind the

Biehl memorial. While filling my car in Cape Town one day it occurred to me that gas stations in the city really don't need my business. There are plenty of Capetonians and tourists filling their tanks in the city. People need to be spending money in the townships if there is ever going to be job creation there, so I decided to patronize businesses in Guguletu. Since I'm also always looking for ways to save time, frequenting the Caltex station would allow my guests to see the monument while my car was being filled with gas.

There are no self-service gas stations in South Africa, and if you think about it, this makes sense. In a country with massive unemployment, having station attendants is another way to create jobs. Since it is customary to tip attendants, their attention to your car is complete.

Nearly every week, with a visitor from the United States in tow, I would pull up to the pump at the Guguletu Caltex. On this particular visit, three attendants swooped down on the vehicle. One began filling the tank, another asked to check the air, water, and oil, while a third began washing the windshield. I pointed my friend in the direction of the Biehl memorial about fifteen yards from the station, and I stood halfway between my car and my guest. I was being overly cautious, I know, but crime can happen in a split second. My friend was taking photos of the monument, making her and her camera easy targets for a quick run-by mugging. At the same time, an unlocked and unattended car, even at a gas station, could prove too inviting an opportunity for a carjacker to pass up. I was trying to keep an eye on both my guest and my car. It was a windy day in Guguletu. A southeaster had come in to blow all the pollution in the city out to sea. Thankfully, the wind also sent my friend quickly back inside the car, where I could easily keep an eye on both vehicle and guest as the attendant continued to fill the tank with gas.

A full-service gas station means there is no quick stop to get fuel, but this particular stop at the Caltex was taking an especially long time. As I watched while the tank of my car was slowly being filled with gas, a few other cars sped in and out of the station. These were township cabs coming in for a few rands' worth of gas. Most of these cabs in the township are owned by entrepreneurial people who somehow get enough money together to buy a beater of a car that they use to transport fares around the townships for a small cost. These vehicles run as much on prayer as they do on gasoline. Their owners don't have enough money to fill the tank of their cars, so consequently they are in and out of gas stations all day, putting in small amounts of gas between fares. As these cabs sped in and out of the Caltex, I continued to wait as the attendant slowly topped off my tank, determined to get every possible tenth of a rand of fuel into it.

I was beginning to grow impatient when a man appeared from behind me. He didn't introduce himself. Instead, he began asking me questions about where I came from and what was I doing in Guguletu. In situations like these, I'm immediately suspicious. I quickly let the man know that I was not lost, that I worked down the street at the community center, and that I intentionally came to this station. I introduced myself and asked him who he was. His name was Zain Simon, the owner of the Caltex.

Clearly, Mr. Simon was curious about this white man who was filling his car at a station in Guguletu. I was just as curious about Mr. Simon.

Mr. Simon had not heard of the community center where I worked. He asked me what kind of programs happened there, and seemed especially interested in those addressing the needs of children. "Come inside, I have something for you." I followed Mr. Simon in through the thick gates that protect his station, while trying to again keep an eye on my friend sitting patiently in the car.

Mr. Simon had been running promotions to try to draw new customers to his station. The day before my visit, he had been giving away toys: small plastic cars and trucks in bold primary colors and plastic viewmasters — the toy most people my age fondly remember from our own childhoods. Each viewmaster came with one circle of images that children could click through to see a different story told through cartoon images. There were only a few viewmasters in the box Mr. Simon showed me, but there still had to be thirty small plastic toys. Mr. Simon said he wanted the children at the community center to have the remaining toys. He said businesses have a responsibility to give back to their community, no matter where that community is.

This visit to the Caltex station was on the Friday of the most frustrating week I had experienced in Guguletu. Scheduled meetings were canceled at the last minute. Emergencies had replaced the work I had hoped to do. I was tired and felt stymied by the lack of progress I was making at the community center. I feared I was becoming cynical about my work. I needed a break from the townships.

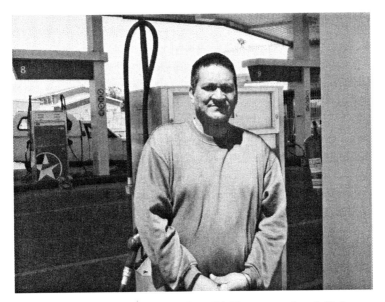

On the site where American Amy Biehl was murdered, Zain Simon performs an act of kindness.

Then, in truly the most unexpected place—a gas station located near the spot where Amy Biehl was murdered—an act of kindness and generosity occurred. A few plastic toys transformed my week. Mr. Simon's simple donation of leftover toys from a corporate promotion was all I needed to restore my confidence in people. The gesture confirmed my long-standing belief, a belief that had begun to falter during this terrible week, that most people are basically good and when they hear of a need, they respond to it.

I left the Caltex station with a full tank of gas, a box full of toys, and renewed energy to return to work in Guguletu the following week.

BEREAVEMENT CALL

With a sweep of her hand, an American friend discounted our work in South Africa by saying, "People there just don't respect life the same way we do in the U.S." Maybe she would think differently had she been with us in the townships on one particular day.

Along with some friends from America, I had gone to Guguletu one Sunday morning to attend services in Reverend Spiwo Xapile's Presbyterian church. Minutes after the service began it was disrupted by the explosive wailing of a woman who was quickly led from the church, sobbing all the way. Two hours later the service ended, and we discovered that the woman had just learned that a family member had died of AIDS earlier in the day. Another two hours would find us sitting in the room where the woman's relative had died.

Reverend Xapile drove us around Guguletu following the service that morning. Eventually he stopped his car in front of a home where people literally overflowed from the house, into the yard and street. We had come, the Reverend said, to make a bereavement call. The Americans all told the pastor that he should pay his respects and we would wait in the car, but Reverend Xapile would hear none of it.

We got out of the car and followed the minister as he snaked his way through the mourners, into the house and the tiny, sweltering bedroom where the young woman had died. The deceased woman's mother slouched on a mattress on the floor, surrounded and supported by other women, covered with blankets in the summer heat, a box of tissues on her lap.

We extended our condolences to the women on the bed and the other mourners, who sat on benches that lined the walls of the bedroom. The mourners offered us their chairs or spots on the benches, and we sat and listened as their minister spoke and prayed in Xhosa with the family. After the prayer, the dead woman's father rose from his seat and acknowledged the words of the *umfundisi,* the Xhosa word for minister. He turned to us, this group of strangers from the United States, and thanked us for coming to their home to be with them. Then he began to talk about his daughter.

Rochelle was twenty-three years old, the youngest of five children, when she died just twelve hours before in the very room where we now gathered. Her father didn't mention HIV/AIDS. He said Rochelle died of a "swollen heart." Her mother's favorite child, Rochelle had graduated from high school and had continued her education by studying computers. The family could find only two photos of Rochelle to show us—one of her as a young girl in public school, and one taken much more recently but before Rochelle became visibly ill.

Rochelle's father said that he hoped the funeral could be in a week, but it might have to wait as long as two weeks. Rochelle's sister, who lived in Port Elizabeth, didn't get paid for two weeks, so she wouldn't have the money until then to travel to Guguletu for the funeral. Rochelle's father didn't want to wait that long because the family didn't have the money for the funeral, let alone an extended bereavement period. The funeral could cost five thousand rand, a little more than eight hundred American dollars, but the family must also pay for food and drink for all the mourners who stopped by the house, and mourners would come every day until Rochelle was buried.

During our visit we were served homemade ginger beer. Our refreshments would be added to the costs of a death that the family already could not afford. Later, Reverend Xapile told us that casual acquaintances will often call on bereaved families because they have no food in their homes. And people know that there is usually food in a house in mourning.

The Reverend summed up our day: "You ask me what AIDS does to families. It destroys them. By the time they die, the family is finished. By the time they die, all that they worked for is gone. And if the family suffers, the community suffers. With the absence of food, they go very fast. No one in Guguletu can afford the drugs. There is no morphine at the end of life. There are pain tablets—aspirin. What destroys me as a pastor is that it's a very lonely death."

A DOMESTIC'S DAY

♦

I'm sitting in my rented apartment, perched high above Cape Town. Through the living room window, I watch as the day fades and the lights of the city slowly come on, one after another. The pink skies above the sea in Table Bay predict a "sailor's delight." Through the common wall of my apartment and my landlady's flat I hear a recording of Norah Jones singing, "Come away with me . . ."

Dogs are barking. Dogs are always barking in the neighborhoods of Cape Town—a primitive, though highly effective security system. When the dogs stop after a few minutes, I can hear the chattering of birds. Perhaps it's guinea fowl—the blue-headed bird you shouldn't eat in any month that has the letter *r* in it. Or is it that you only eat guinea fowl from September to April? I forget. It doesn't much matter. I've tried guinea fowl, and I won't be ordering it again anytime soon. Instead, I enjoy the carrot and coriander soup I picked up from a quaint market down the street.

Grace, the domestic who works for my landlady, has delivered a week's worth of laundry to me. Everything is ironed, including my underwear. My landlady told me to pay Grace twenty rand, about three dollars, for all the pants, shirts, socks, and underwear that miraculously appear back in my closet and drawers every Monday afternoon. White people here tell me it's best not to pay domestics too much money because ultimately this will upset the informal economy of South Africa. I wonder, though: is it the economy they want to protect, or is it their lifestyle?

I don't know very much about Grace. I know that she lives in Khayelitsha, the largest township outside of Cape Town created by the apartheid government to segregate blacks from whites. There are homes in Khayelitsha that are made of concrete and have rooms with doors, as well as windows, electricity, and water. Perhaps Grace lives in one of these, but it's doubtful. More than likely, she lives in what she herself might call a "shack"—a dwelling assembled from whatever materials she and her family scavenged: discarded wood, bits of corrugated metal, street signs. Inside, the walls are probably adorned with pictures torn from magazines. Old linoleum might cover the floor—or the ground if her house doesn't have a floor.

When it rains, as it does a lot in the winter, water probably comes in from whatever has been fashioned for a roof, as well as up from the ground. Last week it was a record cold spell for Cape Town—temperatures fell below freezing. Thirty degrees Fahrenheit isn't that cold, unless of course you don't have a source of heat. Many people in Khayelitsha burn paraffin for heat. You smell it the minute you walk into their homes. The noxious smell gives me headaches. It's not unusual for the paraffin to start fires that easily spread from shack to shack. Every winter, some poor people in the townships lose their homes and all of their possessions and suffer horrible burns.

Wherever Grace lives, she doesn't live alone. She probably has a child or several children. Her husband or boyfriend may live with her, or a parent, a sibling, or the children of a sibling. There is no difference between immediate family and extended family here—it's all the same thing. This concept of family is extremely attractive to outsiders and an important part of the Xhosa culture. But it does no good to sentimentalize or romanticize it. A large number of people living in close quarters always create stress, even when they're the people you love most in the world.

I'm still asleep, warm in my bed in my fashionable neighborhood of Cape Town, when Grace wakes up in the morning. It's dark when she leaves her home in Khayelitsha and walks past the homeless people who don't even have a shack. They stand over the fires they have lighted in old oil drums, warming their hands. Grace will walk until she waves down a township taxi—a van that carries up to fourteen people and will deposit her at the train stop for only a couple of rand. From there, Grace will board the train to Central Station in Cape Town. She might get a seat, or she might have to stand the entire trip. Someone on this morning's train ride might be robbed. Someone else might be assaulted.

From Central Station, Grace will take another taxi to the closest stop near her employer's home. It might take fifteen minutes. It might take over an hour, depending on how many passengers are in the van and where they need to go. Grace will walk the last two blocks from the taxi stop to her employer's home and my adjoining flat.

My landlady understands the challenges Grace faces

just to get to work in the morning. She doesn't complain if Grace is late. If Grace is still working when my landlady returns from her job in the afternoon, she will drive her to the train station so that Grace can repeat the process to get back home. By the standards of her occupation, Grace is paid well.

A month ago, Grace began to feel ill. She was coughing a lot and missed work. Fortunately, tuberculosis was diagnosed early and Grace obtained medication that she will take for months. She returned to work today, so I will I have clean clothes for the week.

As I've been writing, the sun has entirely set on Cape Town. There is a blur of city lights outside my window and then just the darkness of the sea and sky. I can hear my landlady preparing dinner in her flat next to mine. There is conversation that I can't quite make out. Occasionally, the microwave beeps. I enjoy her taste in music. Billie Holiday followed Norah Jones, and now Charlie Parker provides the subtlest background for her dinner.

The guinea fowl are silent. I assume they have gone to sleep in the trees or on the ground, wherever it is that they sleep. The dogs continue to bark. When I finish my lemon and ginger tea, I'm going to take a hot shower and go to bed. I have a busy day tomorrow.

NAIROBI HILTON

◆─────────────────────────────────────

I'm in that dreamy state of being neither entirely asleep nor fully awake. Crowded into the back seat of one of those small Toyota all-terrain vehicles, I'm between two sleeping friends. We are all exhausted. Days before we had flown from Cape Town to Nairobi, Kenya, and then on to Kampala, Uganda. In Uganda, we had traveled hours into the countryside to meet with women who are struggling, but succeeding, in raising their families and other dependent children in the face of poverty and AIDS. This was the second long day of site visits in Uganda. The windows of the Toyota truck are open, sending a warm breeze across our faces. The gentle rush of air, the constant motion of the truck, and the consistent hum of traffic have a calming effect. Even the Ugandan talk radio that our driver is listening to doesn't disturb the slumbering passengers or me.

At times I think I should break that thin barrier that separates sleep from wakefulness and engage in conversation with our driver. Surely he, too, must be drowsy. But these moments in life are much too rare. I am utterly relaxed. I'm conscious of my physical space, aware of movement, but I'm not really in the back seat of this

truck. I'm drifting alongside it or gliding above it. I am
as light as I have felt in Africa.

A top-of-the-hour news report sends my spirit rushing
back into my body. My head jerks up and my eyes pop
open. I'm awake. A radio report detailing a heightened
state of security for the Kenyan capital of Nairobi has
brought me back to complete consciousness. An alleged
terrorist plot to blow up hotels in Nairobi during the
December holiday season has been uncovered. Travelers
to Nairobi are encouraged to be on guard. After my visits to Uganda and Rwanda, I will be one of those travelers to Nairobi, overnighting at the Hilton Hotel before
catching a connecting flight back to South Africa the following morning.

A terrorist alert in Nairobi is more serious than the
lame orange alerts that the Bush administration subjects
Americans to in its post-9/11 campaign to scare us. A few
days after being startled back to reality with that radio
report in Uganda, I'm at the Nairobi airport waiting for
the shuttle bus to take me into the city and to the Hilton
Hotel. The clerk at the shuttle desk explains the effect that
terrorism has had on tourism in Kenya. The tourists who
do still come to Kenya—and the numbers are reduced—
rarely go into Nairobi, opting instead to leave immediately for safaris at game parks. The economic ramifications
are felt first by the people who can least afford it. William,
the clerk, explains that for a few Kenyan shillings he can
arrange with a friend at the Hilton to have my room upgraded to executive class. I hand him the equivalent of
three American dollars and William calls the hotel.

I'm the only passenger in the shuttle van between the

airport and the hotel. It's a Sunday afternoon and the streets of Nairobi are quiet—eerily so. Or are they? Eerily quiet, I mean. I wonder if this is really normal for a Sunday afternoon in Nairobi. Perhaps the security alerts have jaded my first impressions of the city.

Concrete pylons surround the Hilton Hotel, making it difficult for a suicide bomber to drive a vehicle into the building. The guard manning the security gate waves at the driver of the shuttle, lifts the boom, and allows us to drive to the entrance. A porter takes my luggage and I'm escorted to security, where my carry-on bag is searched and I set off the metal detector when I walk through it. I empty my pockets and have a wand passed over me before being allowed to continue to the desk to register.

The lobby is deserted. There is no line of people waiting to check in. Before I can say anything, the desk clerk welcomes me to the hotel and says that my registration is already complete. My three-dollar gratuity to William also included his friend's preregistering me, so all I need do is present my credit card and sign the registration form.

In addition to a "wonderful view of the city," the desk clerk informs me that my upgraded room on the seventeenth floor (the top floor of the hotel) has two televisions with cable, a living room, and two bathrooms. Because I am an "executive" guest of the Hilton, breakfast will be delivered to my room in the morning at no charge, and I have access to the Executive Lounge located on the fifteenth floor, also gratis. "Your room keycard has been coded to allow you entrance to our lounge," I am told before being escorted to my suite by the porter.

Having never been to Nairobi before, I didn't know if

the streets were eerily quiet or not. I have, however, been in enough hotels to know that the Hilton truly was unnaturally quiet. From the lobby to the seventeenth floor, the elevator didn't make a single stop. Walking from the elevator to the hall, there was no sound coming from any of the rooms, no half-eaten meals on room service trays placed by doors awaiting pickup. Something just didn't seem right.

The porter must have sensed my discomfort. He startled me with, "It's very quiet in the hotel. No tourists in Nairobi. Terrorists." It wasn't the terrorists that concerned me. Being the only guest on an entire floor of a hotel, even if it meant I was in an executive suite, was unnerving.

I tipped the porter a few shillings and walked from the first bathroom of the suite, through the living room, into the bedroom, and then into the second, identical bathroom. Usually, I enjoy quiet. I rarely walk into a room and turn on a radio or the television, but tonight was different. Tonight I wanted noise. I wanted to be reassured that life was going on like normal in other parts of the world, even if that was not the case at the Hilton Hotel on this particular Sunday in Nairobi.

I grabbed the remote control and quickly passed the Kenyan news anchor talking about a murder in Nairobi— some things are the same all over the world. The commercial featuring a Kenyan mother talking about acne to her daughter intrigued me—again, some things are the same all over the world—but not enough to stay on that channel. No to a rerun of *Friends*. No to *BBC World*. And absolutely no to the special on African snakes. Uncomfortable in my surroundings, I did not need to be reminded of my greatest fear and phobia: snakes.

I clicked the television off, grabbed the card key, and headed toward the Executive Lounge. Surely, something must be happening there.

As promised, my room card key also opened the door to the lounge two floors down from my room. It, too, was deserted, except for Walter, the black, uniformed manager who greeted me at the door. The lounge had the feel of an old colonial club for men—or at least what I imagine an old colonial club would have been like at the turn of the last century in Africa. Prints of very stoic and proper British men (and all of the prints were of men; there wasn't a portrait of a single woman) adorned the rich wood-paneled walls. Round wooden tables were scattered around the room, as were sofas and comfortable side chairs. There was a built-in big-screen satellite TV, and racks and racks of newspapers and magazines from around the world.

Walter showed me the buffet of salads, crudités, mini pizzas, skewers of chicken and beef, as well as baskets of chips, pretzels, and peanuts. "To drink?" Walter asked as his hand passed below a bar lined with liquor, beer, wine, soft drinks, juices and various waters—sparkling, still, and flavored. I requested a still water and a Tusker, Kenya's "Finest Quality Lager." With my plates of food, I sat down with a copy of the *Economist* and waited for Walter to bring my refreshments.

As I sat in the Executive Lounge of the Nairobi Hilton, eating my free food, drinking clean water, and enjoying my beer, I found myself thinking less about terrorism and

more about the inequalities and injustices that can sometimes breed acts of terrorism.

An African friend had told me about a faith-based conference he attended at which one of the presenters warned
his audience about creating dependencies by distributing
free food to poor people. The presenter was concerned that
occasionally giving poor, often sick people, food would
rob them of their self-worth and extinguish any ambition
they might at one time have harbored.

Following the presentation, a woman rose to ask the presenter if the banquets served at expensive conferences also
created dependencies for middle-class and rich folks. She
wondered if corporate cocktail parties and dinners had a
similar effect on business people. Did their free meals di-
minish them as people and make them lazy employees?
Why, she wondered, is it fitting for privileged people to receive free food and liquor, yet providing poor people and
people with HIV/AIDS with enough food to ward off malnutrition and possibly starvation should be discouraged?

Certainly, it can be argued that those of us with power
and privilege pay for our food and drink through fees,
business deals, and in any number of other ways. But that
doesn't change the fact that there is always an *expectation*
that we will be fed. Poor people rarely have that same
expectation.

That night at the Executive Lounge, my eyes were
larger than my appetite. After I left the lounge to return to
my suite, Walter would throw away more food from my
plates and pour more potable water from my glass down
the drain than millions of people in the world would eat
or drink on that Sunday.

And there are those amongst us who have never known what it's like to miss a meal or be thirsty, who believe that the abundance in the world should not be shared with others.

I left the lounge and returned to the deserted halls of the Nairobi Hilton and wondered when terrorism might quit taking its toll on the world. Probably never, I thought as I entered my suite, the only one occupied that night on the seventeenth floor, unless we learn how to share what we have with the rest of the planet.

WHEN CHARITY ISN'T ENOUGH

♦

Reverend Xapile asked me to accompany him on a visit to a woman in Guguletu who was just released from Conradie Hospital after a two-week hospitalization. The woman, Nobusutu, has AIDS and was suffering from extreme neuropathy in her legs. She has no family, no home, and no money. A friend was letting Nobusutu stay with her temporarily, but her tiny two-bedroom house— already filled with extended family—simply could not accommodate one more person. It was time for Nobusutu to leave this house, but there was nowhere for her to go. The Reverend was asked to give the news to Nobusutu because the friend couldn't do it.

People in Guguletu easily switch back and forth from Xhosa to English in the course of a conversation, often within the same sentence. There was no English spoken during this visit, but I could tell by the change of expression on Nobusutu's face the moment she realized the purpose of the minister's visit. She needn't worry. She wasn't being kicked out on the street today. The purpose of today's call was to start a conversation about finding Nobusutu another place to live—for whatever time she had left.

NEVER GIVE UP ♦ 89

When Reverend Xapile and I got in my car and began to drive away from the house that very soon would no longer be Nobusutu's home, the first words out of my mouth were, "She can't go to Sisters of Charity."

I told the Reverend that Nobusutu could not go there because this is not a place where you go to get better. This is a place you go to die when there is no other place for you. I can accept a lot of what I see in the townships, but I cannot accept that this is the only option for Nobusutu.

♦

Sisters of Charity, Mother Teresa's order, has a project in Khayelitsha, an adjoining township to Guguletu. A few sisters, with the support of a small staff of workers from neighboring townships, provide basic care to people who are coming to the end of their lives and have no place to go. Seventy-five residents stay in the women's, men's, and children's wards. Come back tomorrow and the number will have changed because another person will have made his or her way to the sisters, or a social worker may have referred someone there, or the police may have dropped someone off. The sisters have never mentioned it, but locals say there is a morgue on the premises—and there would need to be. By the time most people arrive at their gate in need of help, there is little the sisters can do to save them—at least to save them physically.

The patients who are well enough sit outside in the sun. Those who are in bed in the wards are, for the most part, extremely sick. They have AIDS, cancer, other diseases, and serious mental illness. Many of the men are missing limbs. One man is missing an arm and part of his shoulder. "It's all he can talk about, 'my arm, my arm,'" the sister says, clearly tired of the patient's complaints.

An old man with a long white beard is missing a leg, and his existing leg is covered with sores and dried blood. While he is going through the contents of a well-worn wallet, looking for a picture he wants to show us, I try to identify the language he's speaking. I know it's not Xhosa. Since he is white, I think he might be speaking Afrikaans, but that isn't it either. By the time he pulls out a photo of himself dressed as a wizard, I realize that this man who is so proud of his beard is speaking a language that only he can understand.

In the women's ward I meet a young woman whose brain has been infected with HIV. She opens her arms wide and then closes her hands as if in prayer and turns her head. And then she does that same movement over and over again, every few seconds. Unlike the old man with the beard, this young woman doesn't make a sound. She just opens her arms, closes her hands, and turns her head.

When I walk into the children's ward I immediately remember my first visit here more than three years before. On that day there was a boy, maybe six or seven years old, lying with his eyes and mouth open, breathing very shallowly, unaware of anything around him, clearly dying. A friend and I stood by his bedside, shooing away the flies that would sometimes go in his mouth. Today there are two children like that boy I saw three years before.

As I'm leaving the Sisters of Charity that day, I compliment the sister who has shown us around the project on the work she is doing there, and I genuinely mean the praise. I believe there is more that could be done for these patients, but I also know that I couldn't do what these sisters do for even one day.

I ask the sister: "How do you do it? How do you do this day after day and find the strength to continue?" She pauses for a moment and says, "At first you feel, but after a while you don't, and then you can do this work."

At first you feel, but after a while you don't. It's probably sadly necessary that there are people in the world who can get to that point. I just don't want to become like that and I don't think Nobusutu should have to come here.

MOTHER'S DAY

◆────────────────────────────────────

If someone were to give you so much money that you started to cry—for joy or relief or just from the emotion of the moment—how much money would they have to give you?

It's situational, I know. In college, after weeks of eating generic macaroni and cheese, a gift of fifty dollars might have made me cry. Today, I don't know how much money someone would have to give me before I cried. I don't think I would cry even if I won millions in the lottery. Don't get me wrong, I would be ecstatic if I won the lottery (especially since I don't play), but I don't think I would cry.

I want for nothing now. I always go to sleep at night in a bed with a roof over my head. I never go hungry. I can still afford my health insurance premiums. The luxuries in life I tend to want, I can usually afford. In my current situation, a gift of money probably would not bring me to tears. But my situation is different from that of the majority of the people who live on the African continent and who earn less than one dollar a day.

People like Bheki, the young man in Guguletu who dreams of becoming South Africa's greatest in-line skater.

When I wrote about him shortly after I arrived in South Africa, many friends responded with offers of money to help make Bheki's dreams come true. My friend Carolyn wanted to help Bheki, but she also had another request.

Carolyn e-mailed me a message to give to Bheki's mom, Khosi. In the message, Carolyn congratulated Khosi on raising a wonderful son. She wrote about how often mothers go unrecognized for all they do. Carolyn asked me to give Khosi twenty-five dollars, ideally so that Khosi could do something special for herself. Maybe she could buy a new pair of shoes or go out to dinner. In Guguletu, that amount of money could buy Khosi several pairs of shoes and many meals.

Khosi works six days a week at a shop in Cape Town, if she can get the hours. The Sunday I was going to take Bheki to get his in-line skates, Khosi wasn't working. Having never met Khosi, I called and asked her to go shopping for skates with us. She explained that with only one day off a week, she really needed the day at home to get caught up with chores. Besides, it was a sunny spring day in Cape Town, so she would be able to wash all of her clothes (by hand) and they would dry quickly in the sun. Taking a few hours off in the middle of the day could put her behind for the rest of the week.

Bheki was disappointed that the only sports store open on Sundays did not have skates in his size. As I drove him back home to Guguletu, I assured him that we would go to a different store the next day and he would soon have his skates. Even though Bheki's dream would have to wait another twenty-four hours, I had the money from Carolyn to give to Khosi. Twenty-five dollars might not be enough to make Khosi's dreams come true, but I suspected she could use the money.

Bheki guided me past the lines of clothes drying in the sun and into his mother's house—a small L-shaped room furnished with a double bed, a refrigerator, and a hot plate with two burners. Khosi was standing at the hot plate boiling potatoes when we walked in. When she saw me, the first words out of her mouth were, "Thank you for all you are doing for Bhekisisa."

I told Khosi that there were many people in the United States who were assisting her son, and that Bheki and I had developed a plan whereby he would actually earn the money for his rollerblades. I then told her about my friend Carolyn and the message Carolyn had for her. I handed Khosi an envelope that included a copy of Carolyn's e-mail and 180 rand. Before reading the note, Khosi saw the money and tears began streaming down her face. She began reading Carolyn's note and the tears turned to sobs. "Do I thank God, or do I thank you?" she asked.

I would like to say that I had the perfect response for Khosi, but I didn't. I didn't know what to say. I was so taken aback that twenty-five dollars could have such an effect on someone that I just stood there. Khosi saved me by enveloping me in a hug and saying, "Thank you and thank you to your friend."

When leaving Khosi's house I asked Bheki how I could get back to the roads in Guguletu that I know. Bheki offered to ride with me to the main road, and, not wanting to get lost in the township, I gladly accepted his offer.

Ever since our first meeting I had assumed that Bheki had been on his best behavior around me. He had been formal and reserved. As we began to drive away from his mother's house, Bheki's demeanor changed. He became downright animated. Nearly every sentence included the words "Wow!" or "Thank you!" When we arrived at the road I knew would take me back to Cape Town, Bheki jumped out of the car, continuing his chants of "Thank you." As I began to turn onto the main road, I could still hear Bheki through the closed windows of the car, standing on the street. "Thank you, thank you, thank you . . ."

I don't know how much money it would take for me to become so excited that I would stand at a busy intersection and repeatedly exclaim "Thank you" to someone who had merely delivered a message and a gift. But I do know that it would have to be more than twenty-five dollars. And I hope I would be like Bheki—more excited about the gift for my mother than I would be about any gift for me.

WHERE VENGEANCE BEGINS

◆_____

Criminal violence . . . emerges from brutal social experience visited upon vulnerable children who return in vengeful wrath to plague society.

—Pumla Gobodo-Madikizela, paraphrasing Richard Rhodes (from Gobodo-Madikizela's book, *A Human Being Died That Night*)

I spent an afternoon with some of the vulnerable children of South Africa who are going to plague this society with their vengeful wrath in the next ten or twenty years. Today these are kids without parents and families, dressed in tattered clothes, clinging to visitors for attention and affection. Tomorrow they may be burglars and rapists, prostitutes and drug dealers, carjackers and murderers.

In a township near Cape Town, I visited a nonprofit organization that takes in all homeless people and discarded children who have no place to go. Residents can stay for a few days or until they get back on their feet or kick alcohol and drugs—or they need never leave. For many of the residents, this becomes their permanent home.

The woman who takes me through the center has lived

here for seven years. Some of the children have never known any other life. I am reluctant to criticize any agency that is trying to provide service to people who desperately need assistance, but I can't help viewing this particular organization as anything more than just a holding tank for humans.

On the day I visit, there are between 1,200 and 1,300 people living in a compound that formerly was the site of a reform school for boys. There is a married couples' ward where husbands and wives can live with their families in their own dormlike rooms. There is a men's ward and a women's ward. In the single mothers' ward, sixteen women and their children share a single room. Boys can stay with their mothers until the age of seven. After their seventh birthday they are transferred to the youth ward, where their mothers can go to visit them.

Three hundred children, from toddlers to teenagers, make up the youth ward—a block of rooms built around an open square. Each room in the block is home to forty-five children. Some of these children are orphans, others have been thrown out of their homes, and still others have been left at the gate because a mother simply did not have the resources to care for another child. There is no question that living here is better than living on the street alone, but these rooms are cold, dirty, poorly furnished, and house many more children than was ever intended. Each room in the youth ward has an adult supervisor at night, but at 5:00 in the afternoon, there isn't an adult in sight. It isn't much of an exaggeration to call this a coed *Lord of the Flies.*

Two of the young girls are caring for babies. I can't

help wondering if these babies aren't the children of these girls. If these are teenage mothers, the next question that comes to mind is, who are the fathers? If young girls are becoming pregnant in this center, I find myself hoping it's the young boys they are having sex with and that it's consensual. But when we call children "vulnerable," we need to ask in what ways they are vulnerable. And perhaps, more important, *who* makes them vulnerable?

The resident who is conducting my tour takes me to a school. So many children live here that the center has started its own school on the property. I walk into three classrooms. Some of the windows are broken, as are some of the desks. There is not a book or a piece of chalk in sight. If you didn't know these rooms were still being used every day, you would guess that they had been deserted years ago. I'm told that one of the three rooms is the science lab. The only thing different from this room and the other two is that the science lab has a sink in it. I don't know if the water works or not.

My guide tells me the Education Ministry accredits the school. I want that to be true. I want the education at this school to be better than one could think possible given the conditions of the classrooms. Maybe it's a bias I bring with me from the developed world, but I just don't see how that's possible.

What does the future hold for these children? At what age do they decide they want to see the world beyond the gates of the center? How do they maneuver in a world that they have not been adequately prepared to live and work in? What happens when they realize that other children have families and homes and luxuries like phones and iPods. How do they respond when it's the privileged children, who had the best education, who get the best jobs? What are the options for discarded children who emerged from a "brutal social experience"?

Unskilled workers in South Africa can maybe—*maybe*— make a hundred rand a day (about seventeen dollars), *if* they can find work. How much can they get for a stolen car? Or from selling drugs? Or selling sex?

This is life in South Africa for vulnerable children, but is it any different in the United States?

In the United States we tend to invest in vulnerable children after the fact, when they have already expended their vengeful wrath and are old enough to be tried in our courts as adults. We argue over providing poor children and families with adequate housing, nutrition, education, and health care, but we don't hesitate to build more prisons when these children become the adults who plague our society. We install security systems in our homes and cars and move into expensive gated communities, but we say we can't afford to really address issues of poverty that ultimately lead to criminal behavior. We buy handguns to provide us with the illusion of safety and do little to protect the people who are most in danger—vulnerable children.

Americans think South Africa is a violent country. People in South Africa think the United States is a violent country. Both are violent. Both countries must either invest in *all* of their children or be prepared to suffer the consequences: their vengeful wrath.

PARADISE ROAD

◆────────────────────────────────────

I have met scores of people in South Africa and from around the African continent who were HIV-positive. I remember having lunch with a man from Kenya when I was attending an AIDS conference in Durban, South Africa. His wife was dead and his own health was rapidly failing. He was trying to find someone to care for the son who would be orphaned after his death.

There are times when you can help people, and there are times when there is nothing you can do. This was one of those times when there was nothing I could do. I had to tell the man from Kenya that I could not take his son to the United States with me.

"But there is something you can do," he told me. "You can never forget me." I cannot recall his name, but I haven't forgotten the man or his story.

There was another person I met on one of my trips to South Africa whom I *had* forgotten until the day a song came on the radio as I was driving my rented Toyota along a road that follows the Atlantic Ocean in Cape Town. It was a song I had never heard before, but from the very first line, "Come with me to Paradise Road," I knew who was singing it.

I had first read about Anneline Malebo in a Guguletu newspaper eighteen months earlier. The locals refer to Guguletu as Gugs, and Anneline was a girl from Gugs who made it big. In the 1970s, Anneline and her band Joy recorded a song called "Paradise Road," which crossed over to white radio stations during a time in South Africa when radio was not supposed to play "black music." The song was a number one hit. Anneline went on to win music awards, perform with Hugh Masekela and Miriam Makeba, and tour internationally. Twenty-some years later, the Guguletu newspaper took a phrase from the song—"Paradise is almost closing down"—and used it as the headline of an article detailing Anneline's declining health. The paper also juxtaposed two photos of Anneline: one as a healthy young pop star singing into a microphone, and the other one, predictably, a photo of an emaciated Anneline in the end stages of AIDS.

The Anneline I met didn't resemble either photograph. She was too thin and sick to be the diva from the publicity photo singing at the height of her career, but she also didn't have the hollow eyes and frightened expression of the more recent photo captured for the Guguletu paper. Her cousin told me that I was visiting on a "good day."

I had come to Anneline's home because, despite her fame and success, Anneline was now dying and she had no food to eat. We brought a few bags of groceries with us, and even though Anneline was having a "good day," I remember doubting whether she would have the strength to eat what we had brought her.

I visited with Anneline for only a few minutes. During that brief time I could see her energy fade. She stayed in bed with blankets pulled up to her chin, a space heater just two feet from her head. I sat on the bed and told her I was visiting from the United States. She said she always wanted to perform in New York, but that the closest she got was Canada. She couldn't remember if it was Toronto or Montreal, but that Canadian concert had been one of the best of her career.

I asked Anneline where I could buy her recordings and she told me that they all were out of circulation, but now that she was sick, there was talk of reissuing "Paradise Road." How macabre, I thought. Anneline, however, seemed delighted with the prospect of her biggest hit being released again.

When you only come to sub-Saharan Africa once a year, you realize that you don't need to inquire about the health of HIV-positive people you met on previous visits. Usually, they are dead before you visit Africa again. So it is with Anneline. Sometime in the past year she died, and I'm ashamed to admit that I forgot about her.

Maybe that's why Anneline was so happy that "Paradise Road" might be re-released: so that her fans in South Africa, and an American who met her once, might remember her.

MRS. MERRICK'S SISTER-IN-LAW AND I

◆ ───

It's time I come clean on something: I'm a fraud.

The stories I write are true. I journey into townships like Guguletu and remote rural areas that aren't even on the map of South Africa. I talk to hungry people, unemployed people, and sick people. I sit with people infected with HIV/AIDS and take photos of children orphaned by the disease. But there is a disconnect between how I spend my days and how I spend my nights. At the end of the day, I get in my rented Toyota Corolla, leave the townships, and drive back to my apartment in the lovely Sea Point neighborhood of Cape Town.

I park the car in my garage, pass through two security doors to enter the building, and then take the elevator to my fifth-floor apartment. When I'm at my unit, I unlock the iron security gate that provides added security to the apartment. Once the gate is open I unlock two of the three double locks that secure the front door of the flat. I usually don't lock the third one when I leave. An iron gate and two double locks should prevent anyone from breaking into the apartment; and even if someone does break in, there's also the security system that will immediately dial a twenty-four-hour security service. There isn't a "panic room" in the flat, but there are panic buttons strategically placed within the apartment that I could always push in an emergency.

The apartment is big—bigger than my house in the United States. There are two large bedrooms, two and a half baths, a dining room that comfortably seats eight, a living room with recessed lighting, and a separate conversation pit. The foyer is large enough to be a third bedroom.

Along the entire front of the flat is a sunroom, complete with a bar, which overlooks the Atlantic Ocean. All day long, international ships pass in and out of the harbor in Table Bay. Closer to shore, kayakers seem to glide effortlessly along. The promenade between my apartment building and the beach is busy with activity. Families walk along the coast. There are joggers and bikers and children swimming in the natural saltwater pools that are formed by water being trapped between large rock formations on the shore. Most nights I hurry home from the townships so that I can quickly undo all the locks, rush into the flat to sit in the sunroom and watch as the sun begins to set across the ocean. It is not an exaggeration to say that the sunsets are spectacular.

Earlier today I was dozing in a recliner, looking out the window at Robben Island, home to the notorious prison where Nelson Mandela was incarcerated for eighteen years. In the past few weeks I have gotten to know Mrs. Merrick, the woman who inherited this flat from her sister-in-law. Looking at Robben Island, I couldn't help but think of Mrs. Merrick's sister-in-law and what her life was like in this apartment in the 1960s and '70s.

People tell me that thirty years ago Sea Point was *the*

place to live in Cape Town. That's no longer the case, but based on my conversations with Mrs. Merrick and the clues I find around this apartment, it's clear that this was a community of very privileged people.

When I first viewed the apartment, I was struck by how small and outdated the kitchen was. It wasn't until a South African friend visited and explained that of course the kitchen was small because the owner of the flat would rarely enter the kitchen, let alone do any work there. The kitchen was where the black servants worked, and in fact the servants' entrance is still there, now protected by yet more gates and double locks. My friend told me to look out the kitchen window at a single-story building that resembles a barracks. Most likely that building was originally the servants' quarters.

In the dining room, near the head of the table, there is a buzzer that rings in the kitchen. There is also a buzzer in the living room and one in the conversation pit. There is a buzzer by the bar in the sunroom and next to the bed in the master bedroom. Mrs. Merrick's sister-in-law was never more than a few feet from being able to summon a servant to address her needs in any room in the flat.

This is an apartment made for someone who loved to entertain. The bar, the conversation pit, the formal dining room, the spacious sunroom with its spectacular view, the buzzers—there is no way that Mrs. Merrick's sister-in-law did not entertain. What were those parties like in the '60s and '70s? As guests enjoyed their cocktails in the sunroom, did they ever look across the bay to Robben Island and think about Nelson Mandela and all the other political prisoners being held there for decades? If they did think about it or talk about it, were they outraged by the imprisonments? Or did they agree with the government's policy of incarcerating black activists?

As I dozed in the warm sunlight of the afternoon, I was feeling very smug. In my mind I had figured out what Mrs. Merrick's sister-in-law and her friends were like. I had created profiles of people I never met and decided that they represented all that was wrong with the old South Africa. But the reality is that I didn't know the former occupants of this apartment. I had no idea what their politics were. I didn't know whether they were racist supporters of apartheid or if they had been participants in the struggle for freedom for all South Africans.

All I know is how I live in South Africa and how I live in this space.

When I return from the townships at night I quickly park the car in the garage. I set the car alarm, close the garage door, and walk directly to the building's first security door, keys to the building in my hand. At my apartment, I unlock the iron gate and all the locks on the door. Once inside, I immediately lock them all again and, as added precaution, I put the chain on the door. Secure in an apartment many times larger than I need, I sometimes pour a glass of South African wine as I sit in the sunroom and watch the day come to an end.

During daylight hours I spend my time with black people in the townships. Mostly I'm with people who don't have jobs. People who live with eight or more family members in a shack no bigger than my single-car garage. People who experience hunger every day of their lives.

People who are grateful that they have an aspirin to take as AIDS ravishes their bodies.

Before it gets dark I leave the townships, return to a white neighborhood, and lock myself away from the very people I spend the day with. I don't know what Mrs. Merrick's sister-in-law and her friends were like, but if they were more concerned with their own lives and their own security than they were with black South Africans', they probably were no different from me.

The difference is they probably didn't pretend to be something else during the day.

A FEW MISSING BANANAS

◆————————————————————————

The HIV/AIDS support group meets on Tuesday evenings in Guguletu. In September, a regular Tuesday night meeting coincided with one member's birthday. Pat turned twenty-five on this particular Tuesday, and the support group threw her a party. Her mother brought a cake, and members gave Pat small gifts. Amid the joking and laughter, there were also a great many tears. Everyone at the party knew that Pat might not live to see another birthday. The other members were also probably reminded of the fact that they too might not experience another birthday.

I took photos of Pat's party with my digital camera and put the printed images in a cheap, plastic photo album I found in a discount bin at an office supply store. At the support group the following week, I gave Pat the album. She was elated, and throughout the meeting the photo album was passed from person to person.

As I was leaving that Tuesday night meeting two other members from the group approached me and asked when they would get their photo albums. I said that this was a special gift for Pat's birthday, but if their birthdays happened to fall on a night the support group met, and if I happened to be at that meeting, then they also would re-

NEVER GIVE UP ♦ 109

ceive a photo album. That seemed to satisfy one member, but the other insisted that I give her an album as well. For weeks after, whenever I saw the dissatisfied member, she would ask for her photo album. Earlier I had taken photos of every member of the group and given them each a copy, but for this one member, that wasn't enough. She wanted her own photo album.

Like the member of the support group who wasn't content with one picture, there are other people who want more than I am willing or able to give.

The high unemployment rate in South Africa has created some ingenious ways to make a living. When you park your car on the streets of Cape Town, there inevitably will be a man standing nearby who will "guard" the car for you. These men really don't perform any service; their exaggerated arm gestures, meant to direct you into tight parking spots, only make drivers more frustrated and confused. Still, it's a creative way for unemployed people to make a little bit of money. The expectation is that when you are done shopping or have finished your meal at a restaurant or drink at a bar, you will give your car guard two or three rand. Most car guards receive the tip graciously and you drive off, leaving your spot for another driver who will also give a few rand for the privilege of parking on the street. Occasionally, however, a car guard will want more than the customary three rand. He will hold out his hand and say something like, "I would like to have more." I have taken to responding by, "I would like to have more, too," and getting in my car and driving away.

Apparently, the woman I hired to clean my apartment would also like to have more.

I really don't need a housekeeper, but I must admit it's been very nice to return home to a clean flat a few days each week. The woman who cleans for me speaks very little English. She has a limited education and does not possess skills that make her very employable. In fact, she hadn't worked in years before starting with me. She's also HIV-positive. This makes finding work even more challenging for her because some families, especially those with children, won't employ domestic help who have HIV/AIDS for fear that somehow a family member will contract HIV from the housekeeper.

Shortly after this woman started working for me, I began to notice that previously full bottles of mouthwash and soap were suddenly nearly empty. More food than one person could possibly eat for lunch would be gone from the refrigerator. At first I thought that I was imagining this, and I hated myself for suspecting that the housekeeper was taking things.

One day I went shopping and stocked up on food and supplies because a friend was arriving from the States for a visit. Later, after the housekeeper had been in to clean, half the fruit I had just purchased was gone, along with all but one roll of toilet paper. Now I knew that it wasn't my imagination. The housekeeper was—I hate to use the word—stealing.

These are little things. Petty things. A few pictures. A couple of rand for parking. Some bananas and toilet paper. But it wears you down. It exhausts you.

I can deal with grinding poverty. I can handle the sickness and death that permeate life in the townships. I can make the necessary adjustments to daily life to protect myself as much as possible from violence and crime. But at the end of some days, a few missing bananas are more than I can take.

The requests for more—more stuff, more money, the taking without asking—doesn't make me angry. It makes me sad. At times it almost defeats me.

I'm reluctant to talk about this side of living in South Africa. I'm afraid these experiences will reinforce existing stereotypes that people have about poor people, black people, people living in the developing world. I fear that donors will be reluctant to contribute to legitimate causes because of concern that they will just be asked to do more and more. Or that people won't help other people directly by giving a few rand or employing someone, because their generosity won't be appreciated or the assistance won't be seen as enough.

It's easy to relay success stories or stories that hopefully connect on an emotional level. It is much more difficult to show a less flattering side of people. But failing to acknowledge this part of life—the wearing, daily annoyances—is cowardly and presents an incomplete picture.

Of course, the sketches of the woman who wants a photo album, and the car watchers, and my housekeeper are also incomplete.

If I were dying of AIDS, maybe a photo album would be incredibly important to me because I want so badly for there to be some record that I once lived.

If I had spent the entire night on the street, watching the expensive cars of people who are spending money on meals in fancy restaurants, maybe I wouldn't be satisfied with a meager tip either. Maybe I would insist on a few rand more so that my family might at least have samp and beans to eat for a few days.

If I used an outhouse instead of a bathroom and newspaper instead of toilet paper, and I finally got a job working for a man who has three bathrooms and a linen closet full of toilet paper, maybe I would also put a roll or two in my bag at the end of the day.

None of us can ever know what we would do in a given situation until we are in that situation. Fortunately for me and for many of us in the developed world, we will never know what it's like to be poor, uneducated, HIV-positive, and living in the townships of South Africa. Instead, we can dwell on our generosity not being properly acknowledged or appreciated. We can get irritated over the constant requests and demands for more of our money. We can complain about the untrustworthiness of employees when a few bananas go missing.

And then we can go to the store and buy more bananas.

TWO BARS ON A SATURDAY NIGHT

On the night of December 13, 2003, I was sitting with friends at La Perla, an old Sea Point restaurant and bar that is now very "in" with Capetonians and foreigners alike. With the color orange being "the new black" of South Africa, La Perla's furnishings—the orange sofas, chairs, and lights—are back in style. Televisions suspended from the ceiling in the bar showed an endless loop of fashion videos. The patrons in the bar could not pass for the European models pouting their way down the runways in the videos, but it was not for lack of trying. The waiflike women sipping wine next to us showed too much tanned skin with their plunging necklines and exposed navels. The men who vied for their attention drank Amstel Light beer, their sculpted bodies covered with skintight shirts and pants that made their desires a little too obvious.

As is always the case when I see someone who just can't say no to a cosmetic surgeon's knife, I couldn't take my eyes off a woman whose face had been nipped and tucked a few too many times. With a drink in one hand and a cigarette in the other, at first glance she appeared to fit in with the young, jet-setting crowd that La Perla attracts. But the more I stared at her—looked at her wrinkled neck and the age spots on the hands she used for dramatic gestures—the more I thought, "This is a sixty-year-old woman trying to pass for thirty-five."

My friends and I inhaled as much secondhand smoke as the posers who were actually dragging on cigarettes did. We drank our wine and nibbled at our appetizers, about the only people in the bar who actually seemed to be eating anything. We speculated on the woman next to us, who was always getting up from her seat and going to the restroom. Did she have bulimia and was purging the occasional nut and chip she ingested, or was it party drugs that kept calling her back to the bathroom? We decided it must be both.

At the same time as my friends and I were being voyeurs into a side of life that none of us is accustomed to, Lorna Mlosana, the twenty-one-year-old mother of a three-year-old son, was also having a drink with a friend at a tavern in Khayelitsha, Cape Town's largest township. Lorna excused herself to go to the toilet, which was located outside at the back of the tavern. Five young men, teenaged boys actually, followed Lorna, barged into the toilet, and gang-raped her. After they had each taken their turn, Lorna told them that she was HIV-positive. The five boys then beat Lorna to death in the toilet.

Lorna's friend, who had gone out back to see what was taking Lorna so long, was also beaten. The *Cape Times* newspaper reported that "the owner of the tavern apparently saw everything and called to the five guys to clean up the blood in the toilet which they apparently did before fleeing the scene."

Two bars on the same Saturday night in the same city in South Africa.

THE NELLY

♦

Few activities one can experience in Cape Town are as relaxing and self-indulgent as afternoon tea at the Mount Nelson Hotel or dinner at the hotel's Cape Colony Restaurant. Opened in 1899, the Mount Nelson is now as much a manmade landmark of the city as Table Mountain is a natural one. A visit to "the Nelly," as some guidebooks refer to it as, is a step back in time. To drive between the gigantic columns at the hotel's entrance, past the pith-helmeted guard whose only purpose now seems to be to serve as a living adornment of the hotel, and along the palm-lined road to the pink palace that is the Mount Nelson, is to enter the world of pre–Boar War British colonialism.

Table Mountain serves as the dramatic backdrop to the grounds of the hotel. The lawns are neatly trimmed, the gardens well tended, and, I swear, flowers are in bloom— even in winter. Everything is in its place. The guinea fowl that leisurely walk the grass seem to know exactly where to stand to complete a perfect picture of an English garden.

To step inside the hotel is to walk into a completely balanced interior. It is both masculine and feminine. It is the best of Ralph Lauren and of Laura Ashley. (If there can *be* a best of Laura Ashley.) The place has a club feel, but is not stuffy. It is warm and comfortable, but also has an aura that suggests you may want to walk a little taller and sit a little straighter in your chair. The doorman is crisply pressed, as are the porters and the wait staff. You expect to be formally addressed as "sir" or "madam," and you aren't disappointed. Winston Churchill was right when he described the Mount Nelson as "sumptuous."

Afternoon tea with friends is an escape into a world where concerns dissolve away like the scones and cream that melt in your mouth. You sit and talk on the over-stuffed sofas while a pianist plays softly in the background. You eat cucumber sandwiches and salmon sandwiches. You gossip about other guests. You return to the buffet for an-other round of petit fours. You motion for the waitress to bring more tea, and, in a flash, afternoon has moved into evening. The pianist has stopped playing, and the guests for tea have been replaced with others who are enjoying a predinner cocktail. It has been an oasis of good food and good conversation with good friends to retreat to for a few hours.

Located just down the hall from where tea is served, past the exquisite gift shop and the best-appointed rest-rooms in all of Cape Town, the Cape Colony Restaurant is grand and gracious. One wall of the restaurant is a mural of an undeveloped, colonial Cape Town. In the foreground of the painting are steps of a verandah that lead to a foun-tain and there, in the distance, are Table Mountain and Lion's Head. A dark-skinned man in a gold-colored turban ascends the steps of the verandah with just his torso and head visible. Two monkeys, one holding a peeled banana, are placed on the railing of the verandah. A uniformed soldier stands at ease, reading a letter. A cheetah next to the soldier appears to be more on guard than the soldier. Sitting at a table in the restaurant, staring at the painting, you get the feeling that you could simply get up from your seat, walk to the wall, and casually step into the world of South Africa, circa 1900.

The restaurant is all you would expect from an old colonial hotel. Rich, heavy wooden tables covered with white linen tablecloths. Candlelight and, on some evenings, a harpist. You can start your meal with an appetizer of smoked crocodile or spiced ostrich carpaccio. If the Mount Nelson specialties of beef stroganoff or steak fillet are too pedestrian for you, you may want to consider the Bo-kaap chicken and prawn curry, the marsala-roasted lamb, or the spice-roasted springbok loin as a main course. The extensive wine list features the finest of South African wines, including Klein Constantia Sauvignon Blanc and Rust-en-Vrede Shiraz. Malva pudding made with apricots and served with almond ice cream, a traditional South African dessert, is the perfect conclusion to a creative and, as Churchill might have said while enjoying a postdinner cigar, "sumptuous" meal.

The Mount Nelson Hotel boasts that "nowhere are beauty and comfort more graciously combined," and most guests who stay or dine at the hotel would agree. Every time I visit Cape Town, a meal at the "Nelly" is on my "must-do" list. I have lingered over tea on many an afternoon, and I have sampled most of the more exotic offerings on the menu of the Cape Colony Restaurant. I have told everyone I know who is traveling to Cape Town and likes good food to add the Cape Colony to their list of gastronomic experiences.

But no more. I'm boycotting the Cape Colony Restaurant. Oh, I'm sure the food still tastes great. It's one particular policy of the restaurant that I just can't swallow.

Friends from the States, and frequent travelers to South Africa, were visiting Cape Town. Three of us had been to the Nelly before, and we were eager to introduce the fourth member of our party to one of our special places. I didn't know when I checked in with the hostess for our eight o'clock dinner reservation, that this would be the last time I would dine at what, up until that time, had been a favorite restaurant of mine.

Everyone in our group agreed that something was a bit off that evening at the Nelly's Cape Colony Restaurant. The service wasn't up to par, and the food, although fine, was also not in keeping with the usual high standards of the restaurant. Still, restaurants, like people, are entitled to a bad night, and there was nothing so bad as to warrant a complaint.

My friends and I enjoyed the complimentary basket of bread that was brought to the table with our water. We each ordered, had an appetizer and a cocktail, and had moved on to a bottle of wine before the main course was served. Having never had the Cape Colony's signature dish of beef stroganoff, I passed over some of the more creative dishes to try what is billed as a "Mount Nelson Classic." The stroganoff was fine—not nearly as good as the ostrich or prawns I had devoured on previous occasions—but fine. I commented that I was glad I had tried it, but in the future I would return to the more interesting fare on the menu.

Having filled up on starters, scotch, and wine, I ate a small portion of my entrée and decided to take the remainder home. Even if you don't eat leftovers, in South Africa it is always easy to find someone who will. Many times when I take a doggie bag from a restaurant, the food doesn't even make it to the car with me. I frequently meet someone on the street who asks for the leftover meal, or I offer it to the man who has been "guarding" my car as I've been dining. Most doggie bags that actually make it back to the apartment don't get much farther than that. If I run into James, the building supervisor, he always accepts any doggie bag I have with me; or the next day when Lucinda cleans the apartment, she takes the leftovers home with her. There simply is no reason for food to go to waste anywhere, but especially in South Africa.

The others in my party finished their meals, and our waitress came and began clearing the table. When she got to my plate I asked for a doggie bag. As she continued to clear the table she said, "It's city health code policy and hotel policy that we can't provide doggie bags." I immediately felt my back stiffen. In a stern, though I don't believe angry, voice, I replied, "That is not acceptable and will make me very unhappy. Bring me my food." With that, I thought I noticed her back stiffen, and, after an inaudible comment, she left the table.

My friends and I looked at each other. I think there was some conversation around the table, but I don't remember. I was becoming angry and by the second growing more determined that the Cape Colony Restaurant would not throw out an expensive, nearly untouched entrée. I sensed that our young, inexperienced waitress would not be equipped to handle the situation, and I was correct. Moments later, the dark-suited manager appeared at the table and in a quiet voice began to explain, "It is city health code policy and hotel policy that we can't—"

I interrupted him. Although the restaurant was nearly empty on this particular evening, there were other diners near us. Neither they, nor my friends, needed to be party to my escalating anger. I stood up from the table and suggested to the manager that we take the conversation away from the table to a discreet part of the restaurant where we could discuss the issue in private.

I listened to the manager explain why Cape Town's alleged health code policy and the Mount Nelson's policy made it impossible for him to give me my leftovers. When he had finished, I told him that I wasn't just visiting Cape Town and this wasn't my first time at his restaurant. I told him that I was living here and had eaten at restaurants all over the city, including many restaurants nicer than the Cape Colony, and no one had ever turned down my request for a doggie bag. I questioned the existence of this "city health code policy" and informed the manager that even if it did exist, no other restaurant in town was enforcing it. Immediately, the manager backed away from that argument and said that hotel policy still prevented him from fulfilling my request. Besides, he said, even if he wanted to give me leftovers, he couldn't because the restaurant didn't have takeaway containers.

I had had enough.

Calmly, but passionately—heatedly, really—I explained to the manager that my desire for a doggie bag had nothing to do with me wanting a late-night snack or an easy lunch the next day. I reminded him that South Africa has more people living with HIV/AIDS than any other country on the planet and that most of them are hungry. I told him that I was working in Guguletu and that the friends dining with me that very evening were helping to support a meals program for people living with HIV/AIDS in the township. I said I didn't give a damn about city health code policy or hotel policy, that I would not allow perfectly fine food to go to waste anywhere, but certainly not in a part of the world where people go to sleep hungry at night. I didn't care that he didn't have takeaway containers. He could put a napkin over my plate and I would return the plate and napkin to the restaurant the next day. With absolute resolution I said to the manager, "I'm not leaving this restaurant without my food."

The manager caved, but not without first telling me that he would make an exception this one time, but in the future, my request for a doggie bag would not be honored. My anger turned to incredulity. "That's not a problem," I informed the manager. "There will not be a next time. I will never step foot in this restaurant again until you change your policy. Just bring me my damn food!"

To his credit, the manager was always respectful and calm. He apologized. He said he could see that this was an ethical issue with me, and he was sorry to have caused a disruption in my evening. "Sir," he said, "I can see that you are clearly upset. May I bring you an after-dinner digestive on the house to perhaps calm you?"

I couldn't help but laugh. I explained that I wasn't really angry with him or the waitress; it was the Cape Colony Restaurant's ridiculous policy that I found completely unacceptable. No, I wasn't interested in an after-dinner digestive. Just a doggie bag so that we could leave the restaurant.

I returned to the table and to my friends, who were patiently waiting. I said the manager would be bringing a doggie bag and then we could leave. They are good and supportive friends. They never doubted that we would be leaving without the leftovers.

Moments later the manager was back with a to-go container filled with my leftover beef stroganoff. He had wrapped it in a white linen napkin, which I immediately removed and set the takeaway box squarely on the table in front of me. I could feel a flashpoint of anger. Now I had proof that I had been lied to. I suspected it wasn't true about city health code policy, but clearly the Cape Colony Restaurant did have takeaway containers, despite what I had been told. I never lost my temper with the manager up to this point, but now I had evidence of being lied to. I came very close to losing my composure, but I let it pass. I had the food and a small victory.

We left the restaurant and the next day, after cleaning my apartment, Lucinda took the leftovers home with her to Guguletu. I don't know if she ate the meal or if her daughter did, but the beef stroganoff was not in the dumpster at the back of the Mount Nelson Hotel.

I suspect that the real reason the Cape Colony Restaurant at the Mount Nelson Hotel doesn't give doggie bags is that it just isn't in keeping with their sophisticated atmosphere. In a country where people are hungry, however, I not only find that unattractive, I find it irresponsible.

So, I'm doing the only thing I can about the Cape Colony Restaurant's policy—I'm boycotting both the restaurant and the Mount Nelson Hotel, formerly one of my favorite destinations in Cape Town, until they change this policy. I miss the afternoon teas, the walks in the garden, the drinks in the bar, and the sumptuous dinners, but not enough to patronize a business that would rather throw food away than give it to people who are hungry.

HEROES

◆───────────────────────────────

Gugu Dlamini was a thirty-six-year-old health worker who lived in KwaMancinza, a town located near the city of Durban in the South African province of KwaZulu-Natal. She conducted outreach to communities educating people on how to prevent themselves from contracting HIV. Dlamini was public about her HIV-positive status, even discussing it on a South African radio program.

Some members of the KwaMancinza community didn't appreciate the fact that Gugu Dlamini openly talked about being HIV-positive—they thought she was giving their town a bad reputation. Others in town also had HIV/AIDS, but they didn't talk about it. Dlamini had been threatened before, and friends said that she had even been slapped and punched by a resident of her town who objected to her openness. One night in December 1998, Dlamini returned to KwaMancinza, where a mob kicked and beat her to death.

I first heard Dlamini's story at the 2000 International AIDS Conference in Durban. I've heard it referred to plenty of times since then. Some people with HIV/AIDS in South Africa still worry about disclosing their status, citing what happened to Dlamini as a reason to keep it a secret.

At some recent point in our history in America, we became extravagant with our use of the word *hero*. I like to blame Ronald Reagan for this, but then again I blame President Reagan for more things than he was probably even aware were happening during his administration. But it seems to me that Ronald Reagan really lowered the bar on what it meant to be a hero. He introduced the concept of heroes in his State of the Union addresses, even seating his hero du jour next to Nancy in the balcony of the U.S. Capitol, perfectly situated for the camera to cut to the hero of the moment when the president referred to him or her in his speech.

Suddenly, it seemed, a hero was no longer someone who needed to possess extraordinary courage. An everyday act could become heroic, or simply being in the right or wrong place could make one a hero. Death was usually a sure way to achieve hero status. A result of this devaluing of the stature of heroes is that probably all of us, at one time or another, have now been called heroes.

In 1999, a year before Gugu Dlamini was murdered for being public about having HIV, I rode my bike from Minneapolis to Chicago with 1,500 other people to raise money and awareness for AIDS organizations. It wasn't always easy or fun riding a bike five hundred miles in six days in the heat and humidity of a midwestern summer, but I mean, really, it was just a bike ride. There were pit stops with energy bars and bananas, water, Gatorade, and porta-potties every twenty miles or so. In camp at night and especially at the closing ceremonies when the entire ride was over, those of us who took a few days out of our lives to go on a bike trip were effusively praised as heroes in the fight against AIDS. You would have thought we had spent the week rushing into burning buildings to save children the way we were received.

If healthy people who do long-distance biking now qualify to some for hero status, then Gugu Dlamini certainly must be considered a hero. So should some very brave people in South Africa who, after Dlamini's death, began donning white T-shirts with the words "HIV Positive" boldly printed in purple letters for all the world to see. At a time when at least one South African was believed to have been killed for disclosing her HIV status, wearing an article of clothing that plainly announced your HIV status in public was an act of courage worthy of hero status.

◆

I have never done anything that qualifies me as a hero. I did have the opportunity, however, to get a glimpse of what life is like for some people in South Africa who display courage in the simple act of getting dressed.

World AIDS Day is officially recognized on the first of December every year. In 2003, December first fell on a Monday, so most activities were scheduled for the Saturday before to allow more people to participate. Since shortly after arriving in South Africa in July, I had been working with a group of HIV-positive young people to help coordinate a World AIDS Day event at the Zwane Centre in Guguletu. Throughout the months leading up to World AIDS Day, I had also been in communication with the Treatment Action Campaign, primarily through my involvement with Lundi's funeral.

On the Thursday before all of the World AIDS Day celebrations were to occur, a friend from the Treatment Action Campaign's office arrived at the Zwane Centre with a gift. He presented me with one of the famous white-and-purple "HIV Positive" T-shirts and asked if I would wear it on World AIDS Day in a show of "solidarity" with the people of South Africa who were living with HIV/AIDS. I didn't hesitate. Of course I said yes. I was honored to be given the T-shirt.

The days leading up to World AIDS Day were hectic ones. Through the support of Open Arms of Minnesota, we would be distributing food parcels to all of the members of the HIV/AIDS support group at the Zwane Centre that Saturday. A truckload of food had to be ordered, unpacked, and then distributed into 150 five-gallon pails. We had to recruit volunteers to help with this large inaugural undertaking. Speakers and performers had to be identified and scheduled for a special program that would be occurring at the adjoining Zwane Presbyterian Church. With all of the details of the day, I simply forgot about the T-shirt I had promised to wear.

Saturday morning arrived and I quickly showered and shaved, thinking of all of the last-minute things that had to be done before I embarked on the various activities that would keep me away from my apartment until the early-morning hours of the following day. I had to run to Main Road to pick up some food at my neighborhood market. I needed to go to a cash machine to get money for a concert I was attending later that evening.

I remembered my commitment to my friend with the Treatment Action Campaign when I opened the closet door in my bedroom and saw the "HIV Positive" T-shirt hanging there. I grabbed the shirt, removed it from its hanger, and hesitated before putting it on. I never thought, when I so eagerly agreed to wear the shirt, what the implications of this act could be.

In a minute, I would be leaving the privacy of my apartment and venturing onto the streets of Cape Town, declaring that I was HIV-positive. Now, anyone at all familiar with the Treatment Action Campaign today knows that there are thousands of these T-shirts in a rainbow of colors. For some, wearing one has become more of a fashion statement than a political one. To wear an "HIV Positive" T-shirt no longer means that the wearer is necessarily living with the disease. Still, I was uncomfortable.

I was uncomfortable about how people might respond to me and, as I had experienced at other times in South Africa, I again felt like a fraud. Some of my friends in Guguletu knew I was HIV-negative. Would they now see me as a phony? Others in Guguletu didn't know my HIV status. Would they now assume I was positive and see me as more of a comrade? Did any of this matter?

I put the T-shirt on, tucked it into my jeans, and walked around in my apartment. I needed to be going. I had things to do in the city and I had to get to Guguletu soon, but I couldn't bring myself to actually step out of the flat. I knew I would do it. I had promised to wear this T-shirt, but I should have tried it on before this day. I should have lived in it awhile—gotten used to what it might be like to be seen, not for the person I am, but for the disease the shirt implied I had. I remember briefly thinking, "What's the worst that can happen to me?" Certainly, I would not be murdered like Gugu Dlamini.

I did it. Wearing my "HIV Positive" T-shirt, I left my

apartment and self-consciously began making my way to
the market I had patronized several times a week for the
last few months. I intentionally avoided eye contact with
other pedestrians as I walked the four blocks to the store.
The owners of the market, whom I had gotten to know,

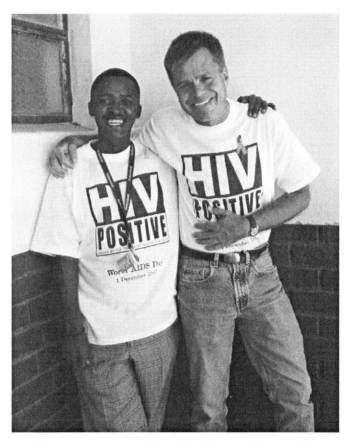

*World AIDS Day 2003 with Michael Matyeni. Later that
day, Nelson Mandela would say, "AIDS is no longer just a
disease. It is a human rights issue."*

buzzed me through the security gate as usual. I thought I caught a momentary change of expression when they connected that it was me wearing this T-shirt, but if I did, it was very brief. They greeted me the way they always had, and we exchanged our usual small talk. They didn't mention my shirt, but acknowledged the World AIDS Day activities by saying, "This must be a big day for you," before I paid for my items and left their shop.

On the way to the cash machine a man dressed in nondescript street clothes stopped me and repeatedly pumped my hand in a traditional Xhosa handshake. Pointing with his other hand to my T-shirt he then disclosed his own HIV status by saying, "Me, too, bhuti." *Bhuti* is the Xhosa word for "brother." Would he still have called me bhuti had he known my true HIV status?

I was eager to get off the streets and into my car to drive to Guguletu and the programs at the church and at the Zwane Centre. Although I didn't know exactly what everyone at the center would think of my attire, I knew they would accept me. And accept me they did. Members of the HIV/AIDS support group shrieked when they saw me wearing the same T-shirt that they were. They asked that a friend take pictures of all of us in our matching attire. American friends have since looked in puzzlement at the photos of Africans and me in "HIV Positive" T-shirts, having the time of our lives. When I look at the photos now, they seem very normal.

Following the program at the Zwane Centre and the distribution of the food parcels to members of the support group, I returned to Cape Town, still wearing my T-shirt, to attend Nelson Mandela's 46664 AIDS concert

being held at Green Point Stadium that night. Billed as
"The Greatest Ever Music Event for AIDS," the name
of the concert, "46664," came from Mandela's prisoner
number when he was incarcerated on Robben Island.

Waiting in the stadium for the concert to begin, we
watched on a jumbo screen as Nelson Mandela and his
wife, Graca Machel, arrived via helicopter and later as
Oprah Winfrey took her seat next to the couple. Promptly
at seven, Beyoncé appeared on stage and electrified the
audience with her international hit "Crazy in Love." The
tone for the evening was set.

Over the next five hours Bob Geldof, Youssou N'Dour,
Bono, the Edge, Angelique Kidjo, Jimmy Cliff, Ladysmith
Black Mambazo, the Corrs, Anastacia, and the surviving
members of Queen entertained the former president of
South Africa and the sold-out crowd in the stadium. So
did the reclusive Yusuf Islam, better known to Americans
as Cat Stevens, who said when Nelson Mandela calls
and asks you to perform at his concert, you do it. Annie
Lennox reunited with her former Eurythmics partner,
Dave Stewart, and brought the house down with a haunt-
ing rendition of "Here Comes the Rain Again." And, for
the first time ever in South Africa, Peter Gabriel teamed
up with the Soweto Gospel Choir to perform "Biko," his
tribute to slain freedom fighter Stephen Biko.

A few hours into the concert, U2's lead singer and
AIDS activist, Bono, took the stage and introduced a
true man of courage, an authentic hero, Nelson Mandela.
The Nobel Peace Prize winner tied together the entire
evening—the name of the concert, its purpose, and the

message—when he addressed the audience. "46664 was my prison number for the eighteen years that I was imprisoned on Robben Island. I was supposed to be reduced to that number. Millions of people infected with HIV and AIDS are in danger of being reduced to mere numbers unless we act. They too are serving a prison sentence for life, so I have allowed my prison number to help drive this campaign."

And then, conveying the message that the world must hear and embrace, Nelson Mandela said, "AIDS is no longer just a disease. It is a human rights issue."

From the moment the 46664 concert began, I had forgotten that I was wearing an "HIV Positive" T-shirt. By the time Mandela, then eighty-five years old, was slowly escorted from the stage, I wished everyone in the stadium was wearing these cotton billboards of solidarity.

For the most part, it's no longer a heroic act to wear an "HIV Positive" T-shirt in South Africa. You see them everywhere. But I remember how shocking it was when I first saw Zackie Achmat and other AIDS activists wearing them in 2000. My shock turned to respect for the activists when I learned how stigmatized and discriminated against many people with HIV/AIDS were in South Africa. That only grew when I heard that a woman named Gugu Dlamini had actually been murdered for disclosing her status. Later, when Nelson Mandela visited an ailing Zackie Achmat in a successful effort to get him to begin taking anti-retroviral medications that would save his life, Mandela himself donned the very same white T-shirt with purple "HIV Positive" lettering.

Thinking about our overuse of the word hero in America, I am more convinced than ever that not everyone a politician mentions in a speech is a hero. Nor is putting on a pair of bike shorts and riding a bike, no matter how noble the cause, an act of heroism. But I have realized that my heroes sometimes do wear T-shirts.

REMEMBERING SIBONGILE

◆———————————————————————

The other day I was rummaging through some files looking for a piece of information on AIDS or South Africa. I
don't even remember now what I was looking for or why
I needed it, because something I came across in one of
those files sidetracked me.

Tucked between magazines, reports, and notes was a
yellowed article from a 2001 township newspaper with the
headline, "Hearty party wish for shy Sibongile." A photo
of Sibongile and her aunt accompanied the clipping. It was
the photo of Sibongile that grabbed my attention. I pulled
the article out of the file and read it for the first time since
I filed it years ago. Then I read it a few more times before
returning it and closing the file. I could file the article, but
I haven't been able to file the memory it evoked.

I met Sibongile only once—on Valentine's Day, 2001,
a few months before her birthday party that was reported
on by the Guguletu press. My partner and I were finishing
up a day of meetings with Reverend Spiwo Xapile in the
townships when the Reverend told us we had one more
stop to make. He said we were going to a local hospital to
visit an AIDS orphan who was very ill. "You need to come
with me," he said, "to meet Sibongile and take pictures of

her. Americans need to see what AIDS is doing to our children, and you will need photos to tell Sibongile's story."

I remember the drive from Guguletu to the hospital as being very quiet. Reverend Xapile was right, of course. If Americans were ever going to understand AIDS in Africa, we would need to connect with the issue on a personal level. I was just extremely uncomfortable with the prospect of taking a sick child's photo. I was steeling myself for the emotions I might be about to experience. The Reverend and my partner also seemed to be caught up in their own thoughts. We drove in silence.

I remember asking one question on that drive: "How old is Sibongile?"

"Four years," Reverend Xapile answered.

At the hospital, we walked down a long corridor into the children's ward. There were maybe two dozen beds in the large room—a child in each one. Some children were sleeping; others were awake and playing quietly in their beds or just looking around the room. A few women sat by the sides of beds next to children. Maybe they were moms, grannies, or aunties. Most children had no one at their side.

Sibongile was sleeping. She wore a child's hospital gown. Her broken right arm, the result of a fall, was in a cast. Her arm might heal, but the HIV-related pneumonia that kept sending her back to the hospital would eventually kill her. My partner and I stood on one side of the bed while Reverend Xapile stood on the other and gently nudged Sibongile awake.

The Reverend spoke to Sibongile in Xhosa. She had that awakened-from-a-sound-sleep kind of confusion. Her responses to Reverend Xapile were so soft that we could not hear them, even though we stood just feet away.

Sibongile didn't know there were two white Americans next to her until the Reverend told her and she slowly turned her head to see us. She was frightened. We both immediately smiled, said "molo," and did what most Americans would do in that situation—we gave her gifts.

We had brought a box of candied hearts and a Mickey Mouse doll in honor of Valentine's Day. Sibongile took the gifts but didn't respond to them. She lay in her hospital bed, looking at the Reverend and at us, holding Mickey, but saying nothing and doing nothing.

Reverend Xapile broke that silence with, "Take some photos."

I took my camera out, made some inane comments to Sibongile about taking her picture, and began shooting. My partner did the same with his digital camera. It was awful. Sibongile didn't respond to the cameras, the Reverend looked pained, and my partner and I were uncomfortable in our roles as amateur photographer-voyeurs. I clicked. My partner snapped. We all felt terrible.

Looking at Sibongile's image in the screen of the digital camera, my partner got an idea. He showed Sibongile the small screen of the camera that displayed the picture of her he had just taken. The apprehension on Sibongile's face immediately disappeared, replaced with a look of utter astonishment. As my partner scrolled back through all of the photos he had taken of her, Sibongile's surprise turned into sheer joy. If a photo had the Reverend in it, she would look at him, then look back at the camera, and then look at the Reverend again. She did the same with photos that showed me in the frame. She would look at the image, then at me, and then back at the camera, simultaneously confused and amazed.

Within minutes, Sibongile had gone from being totally listless and frightened by our visit, to being almost animated. She used her unbroken arm to propel herself into an upright sitting position. My partner would take more photos, these of a smiling Sibongile, and show them to her. Her smile erupted into laughter, and she began rapidly speaking to Reverend Xapile in Xhosa. Now she was playing with her Mickey Mouse doll and eating the candied hearts we had given her. She got out of her hospital bed and sat on a child's plastic chair next to her bed, with Mickey in one hand and the box of candy in the other.

This seemed like a good time to go. Reverend Xapile explained that we needed to leave and Sibongile nodded, never breaking the smile on her face. My partner took one last photo of a beaming Sibongile as we walked out of the hospital.

A few days after our visit, Sibongile was well enough to leave the hospital. Her aunt picked her up and took her home. Sibongile would be in and out of the hospital a few more times, but she was well enough to be home with her aunt for her fifth birthday party, which according to the newspaper article, was a huge affair attended by neighbors, members of Sibongile's church, and more than forty children from her preschool.

I wasn't at that party, but I have been to enough children's birthday parties to imagine what it must have been like. And on Valentine's Day, 2001, for a brief period of time, when Sibongile was discovering something new in

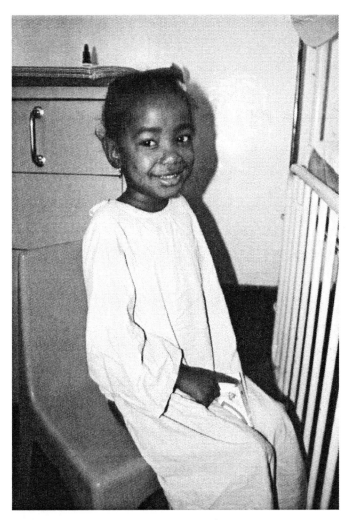

This is how I want to remember Sibongile, as a little girl on Valentine's Day.

a digital camera, I got a glimpse of what she would have been like had she been born healthy and had a chance to have a normal childhood and a normal life.

I know what happened to Sibongile after her last birthday party, but that's not how I want to remember her. I want to remember her as the little girl who sat with her Mickey Mouse doll and candies, waving good-bye to us at the hospital. I want to imagine her as the local newspaper reported—as a regular kid dancing at her birthday party with "her hips swaying from side to side."

SICK IN KIGALI

♦—————————————————————————

It takes less than an hour to fly between Nairobi, Kenya, and Kigali, Rwanda.

It takes nearly that long for me to clear immigration and claim my luggage, even though there is but one incoming flight and only thirty or so passengers on that single plane. Rwandans, with their duty-free bags, clear customs quickly, while foreigners are escorted to a separate room where they pay for their visas. Americans, however, are exempt from the visa fee. My passport is stamped and I join the Rwandans who are already sitting on a motionless carousel in a darkened baggage claim area lit only by a few scattered fluorescent bulbs in the ceiling.

I'm grateful for the visa exemption because I have no Rwandan francs and just a few American dollars. But I'm curious why Americans don't need to pay a fee to enter Rwanda. Certainly it's not because of any support the United States gave this tiny nation in 1994 when 800,000 people—20 percent of its population—were killed in one of the most horrific acts of genocide of the twentieth century.

Waiting for my luggage I become aware of how ill-prepared I am to be in Rwanda. In planning for this trip, I had failed to inquire whether my host, Damascene, spoke

English in addition to French, the language of Rwanda. I didn't know what language Damascene spoke and I didn't know what he looked like, since I had never met him before. I hadn't even "Googled" the keywords "HIV/AIDS" and "Rwanda" before coming here. Although I have read a bit about the genocide, I am not much different from Americans who ask, "Was it the Hutu and the Tutsi or the Tutu and Hutsi who were killing each other?" And so, I arrive in Rwanda with no francs in my pocket and little knowledge in my head about the country I am visiting.

A sure sign that you have left one country and arrived in another is that the billboards for local beers change. The Castle and Black Label beers of South Africa were replaced with Bell and Nile beers in Uganda. In Rwanda, driving the short distance between the airport and my hotel, I notice a competition between Muitzeg and Primus as the "beer of choice" for Rwandans. But there was something more than the language, the currency, and the beer that was different about Rwanda.

The signs of international relief efforts can be seen everywhere in Rwanda, from the UN airplane parked on the tarmac at the airport, to the Red Cross/Red Crescent vehicle we pass on the way to the hotel, to the offices of Save the Children, UNAIDS, UNICEF, the Global Fund to Fight AIDS, Tuberculosis, and Malaria, and numerous other nongovernmental and faith-based agencies that I have never heard of before. Are these hopeful signs of an improving situation in Rwanda, or evidence of the scope of the challenges confronting one of the smallest countries on the African continent?

My short time in Rwanda is to be jam-packed with

site visits to clinics and schools and back-to-back meetings with people infected with HIV/AIDS. I am scheduled to spend one day visiting programs in the capital city of Kigali, followed by a second day of similar visits in the rural area surrounding Gitarama. The sheer excitement of being in a new country by myself causes me to ignore the symptoms that I really am not feeling well.

My first morning in Rwanda, I awaken in my hotel room with a fever. It's more than a fever, really. The sheets of the bed are wet with sweat. In slow motion, I shower, dress, and go downstairs for breakfast. I find a table outside, as far away as possible from all the other hotel guests, who seem to be enjoying their cigarettes more than their breakfasts. When my meal arrives, I just look at the toast on my plate. I take one sip of coffee and know that I'm going to be sick. After a hasty trip to the restroom, I slowly walk to the lobby and wait for my host to pick me up. I have sixty hours to see and experience as much of Rwanda as possible. I am determined that I'm not going to stay holed up in my hotel room because of some little bug.

Damascene arrives on time, takes one look at me—pale and sweating—and suggests that we cancel the day's activities. I admit to not feeling well, but tell my host that we should carry on with his itinerary. As we drive through the streets of the capital—crowded with bicyclists and people walking, not crowded with vehicles—I sit on the passenger side of the truck, wiping sweat from my face every few seconds.

Our first stop is to be Damascene's office, where we will pick up staff members who are to accompany us on our morning rounds. Damascene is driving extremely slowly—

maybe fifteen kilometers an hour. Perhaps he thinks he needs to go slow because I'm ill, but his driving makes me impatient. I know I'm going to be sick again, and I just want to get to his office and a bathroom.

All thoughts of being sick vanish when the truck in front of us makes a quick left turn directly into an oncoming motorcyclist. The man on the motorcycle is thrown off his bike and onto the pavement. His motorcycle goes skidding into a ramshackle produce stand by the side of the road. The vendor scurries to safety as his stand collapses on the motorcycle, and fruits and vegetables spill into the street. The cyclist makes an attempt to stand up and then collapses back on the pavement.

Damascene stops his truck at the moment of impact, and we watch the events unfold before us. Vehicles in the opposite lane do the same. Surveying the scene and the other cars and trucks that have stopped, Damascene says, "We go on. There are others to take him to the hospital. I did it last week."

I'm too sick to even comment on accidents that seem to be a common enough occurrence that just last week Damascene had come upon a similar scene and had taken that victim to the hospital. I'm exhibiting all the signs of food poisoning. And if my self-diagnosis is correct, it's going to be a miserable day in Rwanda.

My first stop at Damascene's office is the toilet, where I throw up. By the time I come out of the restroom, even more color has drained from my face and my polo shirt is nearly completely wet with sweat. "Please, let me take you back to your hotel," Damascene requests. Before I can respond, I hurry back to the toilet, this time to deal with

the other problem. Never have I been so grateful to have
access to a toilet and toilet paper. I realize, however, that
we are leaving Damascene's office and going into the field,
into some of the poorest neighborhoods of urban Kigali.
I suspect that this might be the last bathroom I will see
for some time. I put what remains of a roll of toilet paper
into my shoulder bag and set off with Damascene and his
staff for the first of a daylong series of visits that have been
arranged for me.

Once off the main road of Kigali, some of the side
streets going up the mountains become nearly impossible
to ascend, even with four-wheel drive. The dirt roads have
been deeply rutted by years of heavy rain. What started
as potholes have become craters. Ours is the only vehicle
on the street, and Damascene successfully gets around
the ditches, ruts, and holes, while simultaneously avoid-
ing the flow of people descending the mountain, much
as water must flood down this very street every spring.
Unlike South Africa, almost everyone on the street looks
into the vehicle at me. Even with all of the relief workers
in Rwanda, a white face draws attention here—at least in
this Kigali slum.

Our first visit is to a health care facility that is more than
a clinic, but less than a hospital. It's called a dispensary,
and a doctor there dispenses treatments and medicines—at
least as much as is available of both. A dozen women—
only women—wait patiently with their children to see the
doctor. None of them says a word. Occasionally, one will
glance over at our group of visitors, but mostly they sit in
silence, staring at the doctor's door, waiting for it to open.

The walls of the dispensary are covered with posters

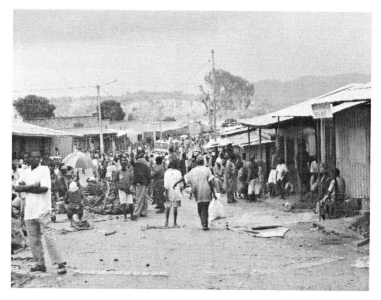

Rwanda. The world turned away during the genocide. Will it do the same as HIV/AIDS ravages the country?

about AIDS, malaria, and tuberculosis. The doctor comes from her office to greet me. Damascene serves as a translator and explains that the dispensary serves people with all of the diseases shown on the walls, as well as typhoid, respiratory infections, and worms. Worms and malaria are the most common ailments.

The doctor shows me the men's ward and the women's ward. They aren't wards, really; they are small rooms that each holds three beds. A thin mattress, flattened by all of the patients who had lain there before, covers each wooden bed frame. There is just enough space between each bed for a person to stand. There isn't room enough for even a chair for a guest or family member to sit next to a bedridden patient.

I stand next to the woman in the bed nearest the open, screenless window. The woman's head rests on the wooden frame of the bed. There are no pillows in the dispensary. She looks like all of the AIDS-ravaged images we see of Africans on those rare occasions when network television reports on AIDS in Africa, or when *Time* or *Newsweek* deigns to feature a cover story on AIDS. I notice the IV inserted in a vein in her hand, and I follow the tube as it leads to a plastic bag filled with a yellow fluid that hangs from a single nail in the wall. On the bag is the word "malaria."

Damascene notices me looking at the bag on the wall and says, "Everyone here has malaria." It's not true, of course, but his comment speaks to the extent of the disease. This woman, who reminds me of one of those rare photos I once saw in a *Time* magazine story on AIDS, is going to recover from malaria, this time. She is receiving better care at this private dispensary than she would have in the public hospitals of Kigali, and the few francs that her treatment costs will be paid by the nonprofit agency my hosts work for.

The young doctor and Damascene continue to discuss the woman's condition in French. I interrupt them. I'm going to be sick again, and the doctor quickly escorts me to an examination room that has a toilet—the only toilet in the entire dispensary. I rush into the exam room where a man sits on the metal exam table, his foot covered with bloody bandages. There's not a separate restroom. The toilet is along the wall in the open exam room. Still standing,

I start to vomit as I lean toward the toilet. As I kneel on the floor to continue retching, I become aware of an overwhelming stench coming from the toilet. It is filled with urine and excrement, and I realize that those same contents are on the floor I'm kneeling on. If I weren't already sick, the toilet probably would make me so.

I can hear the patient with the bandaged foot hobbling out of the exam room, and I'm relieved to be alone. I can't imagine what this man has seen in Rwanda in his young life, but I'm quite certain that he has never seen a white man vomiting before.

As soon as this latest wave of nausea passes, I try to flush the toilet and immediately understand why it is full of human waste. There is no running water in the dispensary, or at least not in this part of the dispensary. The filth simply accumulates in the toilet. The smell forces me away, and I find a spot on the floor that looks a bit cleaner than the area around the stool. I sit down with my back to the wall and wait for the new round of fever to subside.

Sometimes opportunities arise from the most difficult of situations. Although the entire dispensary is small, this examination room was not included in my tour. I would have missed it had I not become ill. Maybe my hosts weren't going to show me the room because there was a patient in it, or maybe it was because of the condition of the room. Either way, I now have the chance to sit and really look at a medical examination room in Rwanda.

A few medical instruments are scattered helter-skelter on a small table. There is a two-door metal cabinet that I want to open to investigate its contents, but am simply too tired to do so. With the patient gone, the stainless steel examination table is bare, except for a piece of blood-ied gauze. A trashcan next to the table is overflowing with paper and more soiled bandages. Additional bloody rags encircle the can on the floor. In South Africa, I have had numerous conversations with health workers about their concern for properly disposing of medical waste. In Rwanda, at least at this dispensary, medical waste removal seems the least of the concerns.

For a brief moment I feel like I'm quickly becoming immersed in a travel horror story. I'm alone in Rwanda. No one, anywhere, really knows where I am. I have known one person in this country for all of twelve hours. I don't speak French. I'm sick, getting weaker by the hour, and can already feel myself becoming dehydrated. Worse than that, I'm in what is considered to be an excellent, private, medical care facility, and I'm sitting next to the only toilet in the building, which is nearly overflowing with urine and feces, and I'm staring at bloody bandages on the floor.

I'm fairly certain that I have food poisoning and that I will be feeling better in twenty-four hours, but there is just the slightest concern that keeps popping into my head. What if it isn't food poisoning? What if it's some-thing else? Looking around at the options for medical care, I decide that if it is something else that's wrong with me, then, well, I'm screwed.

Somehow, I pull myself up from the floor. I search my bag for a package of Listerine mints—the wafer-thin mouthwash strips that you gently pull from their plas-tic case and let dissolve on your tongue and the roof of your mouth. I have served these—like an oral hygiene communion—to hundreds of Africans during my journey. I always make sure I have a few packs with me because I have found that most Africans have never experienced this latest trend in breath fresheners from the developed world, and most people with whom I "break mints" love them as much as I do.

Today, however, I won't be handing these mints out willy-nilly in Kigali. I place strip after strip on my tongue, hoping to rid my mouth of the taste of vomit. It doesn't work. Rather, the lingering taste of vomit, combined with half a dozen mouthwash strips, begins to make me nauseous again. I put the mints in my pocket and walk out of the examination room.

Damascene, along with the doctor and the man with the injured foot, are waiting outside the door. This time Damascene doesn't ask if I want to return to my hotel. Instead he says, "The doctor is wondering if you have been taking your malaria medication." When I nod affirmatively he says, "Good, then it can't be malaria that's wrong with you," and we continue our tour.

As the doctor looks for the key to a locked door, Damascene explains that the dispensary is fortunate to have its own laboratory where the doctor can run tests. It's the key for the lab that the doctor is searching for. When she finds it, she opens the door and invites me to enter her laboratory, which is the size of a small walk-in closet. Unlike the exam room, the lab is spotless. Keeping it clean, however, should not be too much of a task since the entire lab consists of one wooden table and a single microscope. A spiral notebook lies open on the table, filled with handwritten information about each patient. A blood sample between two glass slides waits to be viewed under the microscope.

That's all there is to the lab. A table, two chairs, a notebook, a microscope, and some glass slides. Seeing no other supplies, I ask the doctor if she at least has medical exam gloves. She shakes her head no. Damascene tells her in French that I have brought gloves that she may have. For the first time during my visit, the doctor's face lightens. She shakes my forearm vigorously, saying, "Merci beaucoup, monsieur. Merci beaucoup."

The final stop on my tour is to the pharmacy that adjoins the main building of the dispensary. I don't know all of the names of the drugs, but I'm relieved to see the shelves full of medications and bandages. The doctor can write a prescription in the dispensary, and the patient can simply walk a few steps to the pharmacy and receive the pills that have been ordered. Again, the agency that my host works for will pay for prescriptions for their beneficiaries. I don't know how others afford it, however, and I'm too sick to ask. I've stopped asking questions. Stopped taking pictures. Stopped taking notes. I'm trying to absorb it all, but my own illness is preventing me from engaging with people who are all much sicker than I am, but aren't exhibiting obvious symptoms like I am.

We leave the pharmacy and return to the truck, where I give the doctor a few boxes of exam gloves and say "au revoir." As our vehicle begins its descent down the red dirt mountain road, I search my shoulder bag for a Cipro pill, certain that I threw up the one I had taken earlier in the morning. In a pocket of my bag I find my Cipro; as well as my antimalarial medication, Malarone; Valtrex, to prevent cold sores; Lortadine for hay fever; Nasacort nasal spray; an EpiPen should I be stung by a bee; both Advil and Tylenol; as well as a travel-size bottle of Purel antiseptic hand sanitizer. My yellow International Certificate of Vaccination, detailing my shots for hepatitis, polio, yellow fever, and tetanus, is in the same pocket. I am my own walking pharmacy.

I manage to make it to three more site visits this particular day—vomiting in front of curious Rwandans at all of them—before finally succumbing to my illness and being taken back to my hotel. After a nap and a cool bath, the nausea begins to lessen and my fever breaks. I call room service and order three bottles of Sprite, two liters of water, sorbet, and a baguette. I find yet another brown, white-capped bottle in my luggage, this one containing Ambien. I take a sleeping pill and go to bed with the hope that I will be better in the morning and can continue on with more site visits in Rwanda the next day.

I sleep for eight hours that night and awake feeling a little weak, but well enough to return to the field. While I slept, more than 5,500 people in the world who did not have access to the education, medical care, and medications that I do, died of AIDS, malaria, and tuberculosis.

Afternote

The woman I met at the dispensary in Kigali who was receiving an intravenous treatment for malaria reminded me of a photograph of a woman I had seen in a 2001 cover story *Time* magazine did on AIDS. The woman featured in the magazine was being lifted from a wheelchair. Her body was emaciated; her head was all teeth, eyes, and cheekbones. The caption read: "Last Trip: A 28-year-old woman leaves her three children to enter a home for dying AIDS patients." The photo, like so many pictures taken of people dying of AIDS, was in black and white. It's strange, but when I think of that woman in the dispensary in Kigali, I remember the scene in black and white, even though there was color in the room, of course.

That *Time* article was excellent. It would later be required reading for a human rights course I took at Harvard. Not all press coverage of AIDS in Africa has been so positive, however.

In July of 2000, I was returning from the international AIDS conference in Durban, South Africa, and had to make a connecting flight through Johannesburg. At a gift shop in the Johannesburg airport, I picked up a copy of the international edition of *Newsweek*. The cover story featured a photo of four young South Africans in silhouette, with the headline, "In the Shadow of AIDS: The Plague's Devastating Toll on Africa's Youth." I devoured the article before even boarding the plane to return to the United States. I was ecstatic that the AIDS conference had garnered this much media attention. Maybe, I thought, attitudes in the developed world toward people living with HIV/AIDS in Africa would start to change and the AIDS pandemic would finally register with Americans as a major issue.

When my flight landed in Minneapolis, I went to another gift shop in the airport to purchase additional copies of *Newsweek*. The story that appeared on page 12 of the international edition of the magazine was buried on page

30 of the American edition. The silhouetted image of the four young South Africans that graced the cover of the international edition had been replaced with a caricature of Harry Potter. The headline, "In the Shadow of AIDS," had been replaced with a banner sure to sell more copies in the United States: "Here's Harry: Behind the Fastest-Selling Book in History."

While the real-life AIDS story received three pages of copy in the U.S. edition of *Newsweek,* a fictional character, Harry Potter, got five pages of coverage, plus an additional five pages of an "exclusive book excerpt" and a one-page column written by Anna Quindlen. The Harry Potter article reported that at that point, July 17, 2000, the first three J. K. Rowling books had earned approximately $480 million.

Harry Potter was generating more money than the U.S. was contributing toward international AIDS efforts, and it was garnering far more media attention than the toll AIDS was taking on poor people around the world.

As I paid for my American version of *Newsweek,* the clerk said, "Welcome home." She needn't have reminded me. Looking at the magazine I had purchased in South Africa and the one that I had just bought, it was very clear to me that I was back in the United States.

DIFFICULT SITUATIONS

◆――――――――――――――――――――――――――――

"What's the most difficult situation you have faced in South Africa?"

After "Are you safe there?" and "What's the food like?" I am asked this question more than any other. Usually I explain that I haven't encountered any situation especially challenging, but when a friend visiting from the States asked me the question again—"What's the most difficult situation you have faced here?"—the response that came out of my mouth surprised me.

Nombulelo is as sick as anyone I have seen in the townships. She's sicker than some people I met who have already died. HIV/AIDS has left her blind. Thrush has made it difficult for her to swallow, which has contributed to the wasting and weakness that makes it impossible for her to get out of bed without assistance. The shingles that cover her body are obviously painful.

Nombulelo's elderly mother cares for her grown daughter as she did when Nombulelo was a baby; the only difference is that the mother is now old and in need of someone to look after her, rather than caring for a dying adult child. The mother encourages her daughter to eat, but her attempts are not usually successful. She tries to get Nombulelo to the outdoor toilet in time, but between Nombulelo's diarrhea and her mother's slowed pace, she is often too late. Nombulelo's sister, who also lives in the house, spends most of her time trying to keep Nombulelo's clothes clean. She washes the soiled clothes and bed linens in a basin in the backyard and hangs them in the hot African sun to dry.

At night, the old mother sleeps with Nombulelo in the only bed in the only bedroom in this two-room house. The other adult daughter, the one who spends her days doing laundry, sleeps on the floor at the foot of the bed. Nombulelo has two children who, like their aunt, sleep on the floor by the side of the bed. When Nombulelo needs to go to the bathroom in the middle of the night, everyone has to get up to assist the mother and to clear a path for the mother and her blind daughter. Again, by the time everyone has gotten up from the floor and helped Nombulelo and her mother out of bed, it's usually too late. Nombulelo's clothes and the bedclothes need to be changed before the family can go back to sleep. Everyone in this tiny home is exhausted.

Nombulelo is too sick to work. The other adult daughter needs to assist in the care of her dying sister and consequently quit her job. The mother is too old to work. The entire family of three adults and two children try to live on the matriarch's old-age pension of less than $100 a month. There is almost no food in the house. There are also no medications for Nombulelo—no anti-retrovirals for HIV/ AIDS, no antibiotics for thrush, no acyclovir for shingles, not even an aspirin to alleviate some of her pain. AIDS has broken another African family.

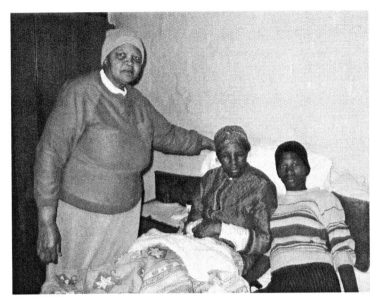

HIV/AIDS takes a toll on three generations of African women. Mabel cares for her grown daughter as she is dying, and for her granddaughter, who will soon be motherless.

But this is only background information. Nombulelo's story is more the rule than the exception for people trying to live with HIV/AIDS in the townships of South Africa. This is not what I found difficult.

Two weeks after my first visit to Nombulelo's family I returned to their house with a bag of groceries—chicken, samp, rice, butter, cooking oil, carrots, potatoes—enough food for the entire family, at least for a couple of days. Nombulelo wasn't there. She had been taken to a hospital in Cape Town because, in addition to her other ailments, she now had tuberculosis.

I asked Nombulelo's mother questions that I was quite certain I knew the answers to. I asked if she had been able to visit her daughter. "No" was the response I was anticipating and also the answer I got. It could cost as much as three dollars for bus fare to and from the hospital, and there is no money for that. The mother has to wait to see her daughter, she said, until Nombulelo gets well and returns home. Everyone standing in the kitchen of this tiny home, including Nombulelo's twelve-year-old daughter, Ntombizanele, knows that Nombulelo is not returning home. But even this is not the difficult part of this situation.

It was a Wednesday morning when I visited the family, and after being in the house for a few minutes I realized that Ntombizanele was standing next to me. I asked her why she wasn't in school. "I was sent home yesterday because my black shoes are broken."

In South Africa, children wear school uniforms, and appropriate shoes are part of that uniform. Ntombizanele's well-worn black shoes had broken—again. The day before she had worn her only other shoes, her sneakers, to school. She was told to go home and not return until she had black shoes to wear with her uniform.

I asked the daughter to see the shoes, and she brought me her black sandals. The glue, which had previously held the soles in place, had come undone. It was obvious that these shoes had been repaired many times. Again, I asked a question that I knew the answer to. Why wasn't she getting her shoes repaired when the townships are filled with shoe repair stands? Nombulelo's daughter looked at her old grandmother, who opened her empty hands, shrugged her shoulders, and said, "No money."

I sent the young girl down the street to ask the nearest cobbler how much it would cost to fix a pair of shoes that should have been thrown away long ago. She returned with the answer. "Ten rand." And this is the most difficult part of the story for me. Less than a dollar and a half was

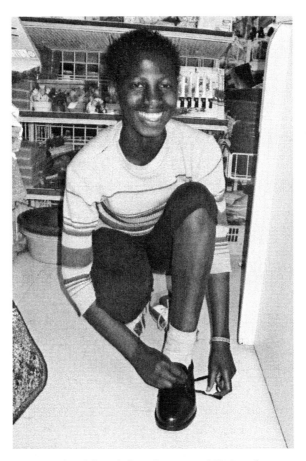

A new pair of shoes brings joy to an AIDS orphan and perhaps keeps her in school awhile longer.

keeping a child from school. I reached into my pocket for the ten rand.

In all of my time in the townships—in clinics, at funerals, talking with people who are dying, whose children have died of AIDS or from violence—I have never lost my composure. I may have been teary-eyed and my voice may have cracked a bit, but I have never lost it. Something about a child not being able to go to school because she didn't have shoes, however, engulfed me in emotion. I put my shoulder bag on the floor and busied myself looking for a piece of paper and a pen. I looked at the floor so that no one could see my struggle to keep from crying. It took only seconds to pull myself together and I don't think anyone suspected what was happening, but for me it was a very long few seconds.

I wrote my name and the name of the community center where the family could reach me. I told them I wanted to know if the young girl was not going to school. I sounded like a typical powerful, white man making demands on a family, but I needed that firmness to mask my emotion. Somehow I think Nombulelo's family could understand that better than a middle-aged white man, crying in their kitchen over something seemingly as trivial as a broken pair of shoes.

So, should you want to know what the most difficult situation I have faced in South Africa is, this is it. It's a twelve-year-old girl who couldn't go to school because she didn't have shoes. But please don't ask.

INSOMNIA

◆

I've taken a sleeping pill, but I can't sleep.

I was up early in the morning and went for a run along the ocean. I spent the day working in Guguletu. I had a beer with dinner, and when I came home from the restaurant I took a hot bath. I swallowed a sleeping pill and read a bit of South African writer Antjie Krog's book *A Change of Tongue*. I shut off the light expecting to fall asleep immediately, but like so many other nights, sleep doesn't come.

I'm house-sitting for friends at their home in DaWaterkant, high up the hill from the waterfront where I ran earlier in the day. Lying in bed, I can look out the eye-level windows at the lights of Cape Town. A nearly full moon illuminates the bedroom.

Geometric patterns—ovals and triangles—are cast around the room, the result of the shadows coming from the security gates on the windows. The same patterns cover an open, blank page of my journal. It covers my still hand holding a pen.

It's some time before I begin to write. When I do, I leave the light on the nightstand off. I begin writing in the darkness of one day and continue into the light of the next.

I'm writing to try to make sense of something that doesn't make sense. I'm frustrated because I can't do the story justice. I'm worried that I shouldn't write the story in the first place. Maybe it's best it remain a secret.

I strike out sentences and paragraphs with my pen. I close the journal and put it on the floor. I try to sleep. I get up and go to the kitchen, leaving all the lights off. I stand on the cold tile floor of the kitchen eating one cookie after another out of a bag, knowing this won't help me sleep. I go back to my bedroom, back to bed and pick up my journal and pen and try again.

This is the best I could do on my longest night in South Africa.

♦

I met Nonkululeko, the matriarch of the family, first.

Nonkululeko cooks meals for members of an AIDS support group at the center where I work in Guguletu. Truth be told, I avoided Nonkululeko for a long time because I couldn't pronounce her name.

I would say to Nonkululeko, "Tell me your name again." I heard her response, but I couldn't comprehend it. I had her spell it, but American English didn't provide me with any kind of a road map to decipher the phonetic sounds of Xhosa.

"My Christian name is Amy," Nonkululeko said. "You can call me Amy."

I sensed Nonkululeko didn't really mean that. Some of my Xhosa friends prefer their English names, but I didn't think that was the case with Nonkululeko.

Every morning around 10:30, Nonkululeko would come

in my office at the center and say, "Kevin, coffee?" She would do the same in the afternoon. After a few weeks she quit putting sugar and milk on the tray when she realized, much to her distaste, that I drank my coffee black. At lunchtime she would bring me a plate with more food than I could eat.

I owed it to Nonkululeko to be able to pronounce her name correctly. At night, back in my flat in Cape Town, I would practice saying her name. Eventually, I had the courage to attempt a pronunciation in front of Nonkululeko. Sometimes my attempts would be met with laughter, other times I would nail her name perfectly, and Nonkululeko and the others who heard me would cheer my correct pronunciation.

Occasionally, I would drive Nonkululeko to the market or give her a ride home from a funeral. Bit by bit Nonkululeko would tell me about herself and her life. Invariably, it would begin with, "You know, Kevin . . ."

"You know, Kevin, I still live in the same house we were resettled in during apartheid. I hated being moved here. I hated Guguletu. Turn left . . ."

"You know, Kevin, 2001 was a terrible year. Both my sons were shot. I thought I would lose them. Oh, I cried and I cried. Turn right . . ."

"You know, Kevin, my daughter, Thandi, comes for meals. She's a member of the AIDS support group. She's on medication. No, Kevin, she is fine. That's my house over there . . ."

"You know, Kevin, my granddaughter is not shy. She's a very naughty girl. She is only shy around you. Stop here. Sometime you will come to my home for coffee . . ."

Every weekday I would see Nonkululeko in the kitchen of the center. When I first began working at the center, her daughter, Thandi, was away in Johannesburg. One Tuesday in the kitchen Nonkululeko told me that Thandi was back and she would be at the AIDS support group that afternoon.

When I walked into the support group meeting I immediately knew which member was Thandi. She looked like a taller, thinner, younger version of her mother.

After the meeting, I said hello to Thandi. She was gracious, but looked away—a bit shy, like her mother was with me at first. Thandi rarely spoke in the group. As time went on, she would talk a bit more with me. She would ask me to take her photo.

Thandi's birthday is December 1—World AIDS Day. A few days before Thandi's birthday, I asked Nonkululeko if she was going to give Thandi a gift for her thirty-first birthday.

"No, Kevin. It's not like America. We're not like you. There are no gifts for birthdays. There's no money for birthdays."

I had taken a number of photos of Thandi with my digital camera. I scrolled through all of them on my computer, found the one most suited for framing, and printed it. I bought an inexpensive frame, and the next time I saw Nonkululeko, I gave her the photo of her daughter.

"Give this to Thandi as a birthday gift from you," I said to Nonkululeko.

"No, Kevin. I will tell her it's a gift from you."

I insisted that this was to be a gift from Nonkululeko to her daughter.

After six months of working at the center I had to leave South Africa and return to the United States. Members of the AIDS support group threw a surprise going-away party for me. Some members rose to say something to me, some speaking in English, others in Xhosa. When Thandi rose to speak, other members of the group began to cheer and gently razz her.

Thandi acknowledged the group's reaction by saying it was appropriate since she was shy and so rarely spoke. It was important, however, that she tell me something before I left Guguletu.

"I know the photo I received for my birthday was from you and not my mother. I keep it beside my bed and every night before I go to sleep I look at that photo and I think, maybe I am someone. If Kevin thought enough of me to give me a photo, maybe I really matter."

On the day I was to leave South Africa, Nonkululeko took me aside and said, "I will say my good-bye here, at the center."

Thandi, and her seven-year-old daughter, Thembisa, were waiting with a group of people at the airport to say their good-byes.

Thembisa was the same shy little girl I had met at my first day in the center six months earlier. She would come after school to get a snack from her grandmother working in the kitchen. Today at the airport, she wasn't wearing the blue-and-white checkered school uniform with white socks and spotless black shoes. She wore shorts and a T-shirt, but she still hid behind her mother the same way she hid behind her grandmother the first day I met her.

"You're not still being shy with me?" I said as I bent

down and gave Thembisa a hug. She shook her head no, smiled, but didn't utter a sound. In six months, if I heard Thembisa speak at all, it was never above a whisper.

Like Nonkululeko repeatedly said to me, Thandi said, "This girl is not shy. She is very naughty." Thembisa just smiled even more.

◆

It had been nearly a year since I had given Nonkululeko the framed photo of Thandi to give to her daughter for her birthday. I was back in South Africa for a brief stay. Back in Guguletu working in the center. Back to meeting with members of the AIDS support group.

Thandi came into the meeting late. Of the forty people assembled in the room, she was by far the best dressed, wearing an ankle-length dress patterned with pastel pink and yellow flowers. A sweater the same shade of pink was draped over her shoulders. Her black hair was straightened and pulled up on her head in a ponytail. Hair fanned out from the top of her head like a waterfall.

Thandi looked great, but it was more than her appearance that had changed. She seemed confident. She crossed the room, took a chair, sat down, and waved at me. She engaged in the discussion with the group with none of the razzing that marked the last time I had seen her in this setting. Clearly, Thandi had become more accustomed to speaking, and the others in the group had become used to it as well.

On my first day back at the center, Nonkululeko had told me that Thandi had a job doing AIDS education and outreach in the community. I was not surprised to hear that people loved her—that some patients insisted on seeing only Thandi.

"You will see her at the support group. She will tell you more," Nonkululeko said to me.

When the hugs that end every support group meeting were over, Thandi came over to me and we hugged again.

"My mother told you the news?"

"Yes," I replied. "It's great. You're doing well on the anti-retroviral medication, you look beautiful, and you have a job!"

"Yes, that's true. Is that all my mother told you? No, Kevin, it has been horrible. I was at work and my sister called and told me to come right home. I said, 'Something is wrong with Thembisa. What's wrong? Tell me what's wrong.' My sister said, no Thembisa was there, but I must come straight home.

"When I walked in the door I knew something was wrong. It was just my sister. You know my sister? No? She has a daughter, too, Thembisa's cousin. Thembisa and her cousin had been playing together, and Thembisa said that our neighbor—a man who goes to our church—had done something to her. The cousin told my sister, who called me and told me to come home.

"My sister said Thembisa had told her cousin that our neighbor had raped her a few months ago. No, man, I said. It can't be true. My brothers already knew and had gone looking for the neighbor. The police found him before my brothers did. Thank God. They would have killed him.

"I screamed and said, no, it can't be true, but I knew it was. Thembisa had changed lately. She was moody. She

168 ♦ KEVIN WINGE

never smiled. She didn't like school anymore. I would be stern with her. I didn't know why she was being so bad.

"I took Thembisa to a doctor to see if this had really happened, and it had. Our neighbor is in jail. He may have done this to others."

I stood listening to Thandi as she told the story with little emotion. It was all I could do to maintain my emotions.

I loved this family. These three generations of strong African women.

Nonkululeko had survived apartheid and managed to raise a family that neither the violence of the townships nor AIDS had killed. In a nation where few HIV-positive people have access to lifesaving medications, Thandi qualified for a pilot program and was doing well. For the first time in her life she was working. And, although HIV-positive, she had delivered a healthy child, Thembisa. Now, this shy, roly-poly eight-year-old girl had become another statistic in a nation with one of the highest rates of rape in the world.

Usually, I would not have asked the question, but I knew Thandi well enough to do so.

"Has Thembisa been tested for HIV?"

Thandi looked away from me and for the first time in our conversation, her voice broke.

"No. I can't do it. I don't know what I will do if she is positive. I thought I had protected her from this. What will I do if she tests positive? What will I tell her? I know someday I will have to take her for a test, but I don't have the strength now."

What mother would?

♦

A long time ago I quit trying to make sense out of the AIDS epidemic. I found ways to disengage from my work and the disease so that I could sleep at night. But what sense is there in the rape of an eight-year-old girl?

Of course, it happens all the time. I wonder how many eight-year-olds—girls and boys—have been raped in the time it's taken me to write this story. But I hadn't really thought about it before. We don't think about these things until we have to. Until we know someone. And then we can't think of anything else.

It keeps us up at night.

And it should.

NEVER GIVE UP

♦───────────────────────

The emotions of grief are universal. Khanyisa Ndlotyeni's funeral was the first one I ever attended in Guguletu. The service was conducted almost entirely in her native language, Xhosa, but I could still understand it.

The community of Guguletu had Khanyisa's entire life to prepare for this day, because Khanyisa was born HIV-positive. In a country where women still do not always receive medication to prevent the spread of HIV from mother to child, Khanyisa didn't stand a chance. Nor did Khanyisa's mother. She died of AIDS years ago.

Photocopies of a picture of Khanyisa are taped to the bare cement walls of the church where her funeral is taking place. The photo must have been taken awhile back. The image is not that of a fifteen-year-old girl—the child in the photo looks much younger, maybe nine or ten. Then again, the white wooden coffin looks impossibly small for the body of a fifteen-year-old.

Even though some of the pallbearers themselves are frail—several wear T-shirts with the words "HIV Positive" emblazoned in huge purple letters across their chests—they have no difficulty in carrying the casket to the waiting hearse. It appears as though one healthy man could have carried Khanyisa to her grave as easily as he might cart a box of books. After her short life of living with HIV/ AIDS, there could not have been much left of Khanyisa.

The cemetery in Guguletu is not a landscaped park with a canopy of mature trees and a carpet of green grass. It's stark. It's the heat- and sun-dried beige soil of Africa. It's flat. There's an occasional marker made of stone, but more often it's a simple wooden cross with the deceased's name written horizontally, and the years of birth and death written vertically. It's like the set of an old Western movie or TV show like *Gunsmoke*, when a character would die and in the last scene the camera would pan to a mound of dirt with a wooden cross sticking out of it. It's like that. Only real.

It's like that. Only instead of one grave, there are hundreds and hundreds of graves. On this Saturday, the cemetery has been extended by another row. I find myself standing next to an open grave with Khanyisa's grave slightly in front of me, and in front of her open grave there is another, and in front of that one there is another, and I know I can make out eight more open graves beyond that, but there may be more. I can't see past the first dozen.

All the mourners come from the church to the cemetery for the burial: Khanyisa's classmates, the community that raised her, and her remaining relatives—one older sister and two aunties. The family rented buses to transport the congregation from the church to the graveyard and then back to Khanyisa's home for lunch. Few people in Guguletu have cars, so the bereaved family must pay for coaches. It's part of the custom of death here.

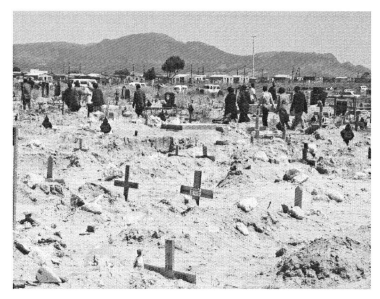

Cemetery in Guguletu.

As hundreds of people try to gather around Khanyisa's casket, more rented buses bringing mourners for other funerals are coming through every entrance of the cemetery. For a moment, I'm claustrophobic. I'm in the middle of a crowd, and everywhere I look, more and more people are streaming into the cemetery. A small funeral band begins to perform at another burial service a half dozen graves away. I can no longer hear what the minister is saying. It's noise. And music. And people. And buses lining up along the road.

Khanyisa's casket has been lowered into the ground, into the dirt. I still can't hear what the minister is saying, but I understand his gesture. He removes the red AIDS ribbon from his lapel and drops it into the grave, onto the white lid of Khanyisa's coffin. The mourners follow suit, removing their red ribbons and letting them blanket the small white casket.

There is a spiritual that I have heard sung at every church service I've attended in Guguletu, at every funeral. The chorus goes something like: "Never give up. Never give up. We shall never, never, never—never give up."

After Khanyisa's funeral, I return to the church. Taped to the wall, along with the photo of a girl who looked too young to be fifteen, is a handwritten sign that reads, "Never give up. Never, never, never—never give up."

"ENKOSI KAKHULU" (THANK YOU VERY MUCH)

♦

I had been warned.

"People in Guguletu are going to see you, a white guy working in the townships, as just one big dollar sign. They will constantly be asking you for money, and if you start giving it to them, it will never stop. The more you do, the more you give, the more they will want. And don't expect a thank-you. They put out their hands, you give them the money, and that's the end of the story . . . until the next time you see them."

White South Africans told me this. Americans with experience in international development told me this. And Americans whose feet have never touched African soil told me this.

I'm back in the U.S. now, having left the heat and sunshine of a South African summer for the cold and snow of a Minnesota winter. I haven't yet adjusted to the time difference. I go to bed early and get up early. The noise from the ocean waves that I would listen to through the open windows in my Cape Town apartment has been replaced by the absolute silence of a four o'clock winter's morning.

The freshly fallen snow muffles what little sound I hear outside my home.

I'm still unpacking. I grab a bunch of clothes from my suitcase, and a tiny child's diary with butterflies and imaginary creatures on the cover drops to the floor. Pat gave me this gift at a meeting of the HIV/AIDS support group at the community center. Pat had been moved by something she heard in a church sermon the Sunday before. At the service, the minister talked about how rarely we tell people we love them. Pat stood up at the support group meeting and said that there was a member of the group that she wanted to say "I love you" to. To the "oohs and aahs" of the support group, Pat continued. "I want to tell Caven [the English pronunciation and spelling of my name is difficult for some Xhosa people] that I love him."

Crying, Pat told the group that the party we had for her twenty-fifth birthday a few weeks earlier was the first birthday party she had ever had. I had taken photos of the party and given them to Pat in a little plastic photo album. "Your camera," Pat said to me, "makes me smile a lot and gives me hope for a bright future. All people smile in the same language. I don't have much to give you, but I hope this gift expresses how much I appreciate you. Thanks for being you and for giving joy to our lives." I hugged Pat and through my own tears whispered a quiet "Enkosi" in her ear. When I sat down, I saw that Pat and I were not the only people at the support group that night drying our eyes.

"Don't expect a thank-you," I had been told. But, I was thanked, and this was not the only time.

Mary Sili is a force of nature who runs a senior citizen center in Guguletu. If you meet her once, you will never forget her. Mary's father was black, her mother coloured—the South African category for a person of mixed race. During apartheid, the South African government looked at the dark color of Mary's skin and judged her as black. The white government determined that her lighter-skinned sister was coloured. These differentiations based on skin color were important. They determined where people could live and where they could go to school. The irony of labeling one sibling black while identifying another as coloured appears to have been lost on the government of the time.

Mary's parents died when she was young, and she grew up in a Catholic orphanage. Throughout her life, she always managed to find work—first as a domestic, later with Catholic-based social service agencies. She raised five sons and a daughter, assists with the raising of her grandchildren, and is now thinking of volunteering with children orphaned by AIDS when she retires in a few years.

The day before I returned to the United States, I stopped by the senior center to say good-bye to Mary. She gave me an envelope and told me not to open it until I was on the plane flying home. I made it to the gate at the airport before reading her letter.

Dearest Kevin,

I have been thinking of you all the time and it is with sadness in my heart that I realize time is drawing near for you to go home to your family. Bless the womb which you laid in. Your mum has been blessed with a wonderful son. I thank God over and over for having brought you into my life.

Kev, as others call you, I am going to miss you. Please tell your family all about me. I hope I did not bore you with all my talking. Maybe one day we will do something for the AIDS orphans—by that time there will be many more.

I'm sure you must wonder why I show so much love for you and your friends. You must try to understand that never have we been so loved and cared for, even by our own South African people. They don't even know where we live.

Please keep up the good work. Ask your family if they don't want to adopt me as an elder sister. Tell them because of you, I love them all. With lots of love and best wishes. Till we meet again.

Mary

"The more you do, the more you give, the more they will want." Mary never asked me for anything. Nor did Ishmael James, the building supervisor who looked after the Villa D'Este apartment building where I stayed during my time in Cape Town.

James is young, maybe twenty-one. His mother is very old. "She's in her late forties," James told me. James is from one of the poorest countries in the world, Malawi. In Malawi, the average life expectancy is forty-one; so you see, his mother really is old. James left his home three years ago, hoping for a better life in South Africa. He found it in Cape Town, where he lives in a room near

178 • KEVIN WINGE

the garage of the Villa D'Este, and where every day he sweeps and washes floors, tends to the gardens, takes out the garbage, and does whatever the tenants ask him to do.

It is customary, in parts of Malawi, for the oldest surviving brother to inherit the land and property of a brother who dies. The deceased brother's widow also becomes, in effect, another wife of her dead husband's brother. The surviving brother is charged with caring for the deceased's wife and family. That is what should have happened when James's father died, but James's father did not die naturally. As in a Shakespearean tragedy, James's father was ambushed one night walking home to his village and murdered, by his own brother, James's uncle.

James's mother refused to be taken as a wife by the very man who murdered her husband. Her refusal resulted in her having to leave her home and try to survive on a small parcel of unwanted land in a country notorious for drought, malnutrition, and starvation. James left Malawi to find work and send money back to his mother and siblings.

Nearly every morning, as I would leave the apartment building for the day, James would be mopping the floors of the lobby. He would greet me with a huge smile and without ever really looking directly at me, he would tell me to be careful in Guguletu. Some days he would tell me that my car was dirty and he would wash it for me. Whenever I received mail, James would deliver it to my apartment because he knew I rarely checked my mailbox. We talked about his family, about HIV/AIDS, about how he wished he had married in Malawi before coming to South Africa because he is lonely in his new country.

The day I was leaving South Africa, I found an envelope from James taped to my front door. In the enclosed note James wrote: "I would like to say thanks for your kindness, helpfulness and attitude toward me. I still remember all the good things you have done for me."

What were the good things I did for James? I really needed to think about that. I gave him a tip when he washed my car or when he signed for a package. I always gave him a few extra rand and suggested he send part of it to his mother in Malawi to buy fertilizer or seeds so that perhaps she could survive the next drought. After I read the *Cape Times* I would leave it by James's door for him to read. James loves reading, but even at a mere fifty cents a copy, the daily newspaper was too expensive for him. If I had a doggie bag from dinner at a restaurant I would ask James if he wanted it. He always said yes. When packing to return home I realized that I couldn't possibly fit everything into my suitcases. I had a couple of shirts that I thought might fit James, and I gave them to him. You would have thought I had given him an airline ticket to the States, which, by the way, is James's dream.

That's what I did for James. I gave him some leftover food, newspapers after I had read them, and some used clothes. I only tipped him for work that he did for me. Perhaps what James was really thanking me for was taking the time to get to know him a little, for asking him about his life—for treating him, a relative stranger in a different country, the same way I wanted people to treat me during my time in a foreign land. I treasure the note James taped to my door on my last day in Cape Town, but I also wonder why treating someone with basic respect and dignity warranted acknowledgment and a thank-you.

◆

James went out of his way to thank me, but at least for him, he only had to go from the ground floor of the apartment building to my fifth-floor apartment. Mandla Majola of the Treatment Action Campaign (TAC), South Africa's legendary HIV/AIDS advocacy organization, traveled by train and foot from Khayalitsha, a neighboring township, to say good-bye. Because of my impatience, I almost missed seeing him.

It was my last Tuesday in South Africa. I had come one last time to the HIV/AIDS support group in Guguletu, but I was really preoccupied with the to-do list running through my head. I had to disconnect the phone and electricity, return the rental car, pack, go to the bank and post office—seemingly a hundred things that had to happen within seventy-two hours before I departed the country. After a few quick good-byes, I had planned on leaving Guguletu and returning to Cape Town to continue working on my departure. Then my phone rang. It was Mandla saying that he had to see me that very afternoon.

I could never say no to Mandla. Early in my stay, he agreed to take time out of his very hectic schedule to show me TAC's offices and to talk to me about the organization's work. Our conversations went beyond HIV/AIDS, however. We talked about South Africa's Black Consciousness movement, Presidents Nelson Mandela and Thabo Mbeki, access to health care for all South Africans. We crossed a lot of divides—cultural, racial, class, geographic—and became friends. Now, Mandla wanted to talk to me again. I wanted to return to Cape Town and my packing, but as I said, it was Mandla who was calling. I couldn't say no. I would wait for him.

Minutes turned into hours and I was still waiting at the community center in Guguletu for Mandla to show up. I called him and he said he was "coming now." Mandla was always "coming now," but that didn't necessarily mean that he was close to where he needed to be. I waited. I called him again, an hour later, but his cell phone was turned off. Finally, he called and said he was off the train and walking toward the home of a deceased TAC member. Could I meet him there?

I got in my car and hurried to our meeting site. On the drive, I wondered what it was Mandla needed to talk about. I tried to switch my thinking from being focused on leaving the country to being open to whatever crisis or problem Mandla might be experiencing that I could assist with. It wasn't working. My mind was on leaving. Had I told Mandla I couldn't meet him, I already would have been back in Cape Town, ticking items off my list. Now, it was too late. I would find out what Mandla needed and try to get back home as quickly as possible.

Unless you live and work on the frontlines of HIV/ AIDS in South Africa, you can't even begin to imagine the toll it takes on one's life. One of the admirable aspects of the Treatment Action Campaign is that it has managed to create a nationwide movement to address a myriad of issues associated with HIV/AIDS and still not lose sight of the fact that the movement is about people. But fighting for the lives of people you know—not faceless people,

but your neighbors, your friends, and your comrades—
day after day, year after year, is exhausting. And Mandla
looked tired.

"My friend," Mandla said to me, "I'm not well. I've
been to the doctor and I've got this prescription, but I'm
not well. And this week we are trying to decide how TAC
should respond if the government does not begin rolling
out anti-retrovirals. It's stressful. Can you drive me home?
We can talk on the way."

As we drove through the now familiar streets of
Guguletu, Mandla told me more about what was happening with him and with TAC. We couldn't drive more
than a few meters without Mandla waving at someone or
shouting to someone out the open window. We talked as
friends, but I couldn't figure out what the urgency was
to Mandla's request to see me this particular afternoon.
When we pulled up to his house, Mandla answered my
silent question. TAC wanted to thank me and show
their appreciation for what I had done for them. Mandla
opened a bag filled with TAC's famous "HIV Positive"
T-shirts, one of which had been signed by the workers at
the TAC office in Khayalitsha. "Thanx 4 being part of the
struggle," it read.

Mandla and I had not become friends upon our first
meeting. Our friendship developed over time. First, he
called me comrade, referring to the struggle against HIV/
AIDS. Then he called me friend. As he got out of the car
that evening that I had waited hours to see him—that
night when I thought he needed something from me, not
that he had something to say to me and to give to me—

Mandla said, "Thank you. I used to call you friend, now I call you brother."

The next time Mandla calls, I will again wait for him, however long it takes.

I had been warned. "People in Guguletu are going to see you as a white guy working in the townships." I am a white guy. I can't change that any more than Mandla can change the color of his skin. So what? We can still be brothers.

Some people, it's true, did ask me for money. Some even asked for money or food or assistance with school fees or the costs of a funeral nearly every time I saw them. Nombulelo's family was like that, but did they thank me? You be the judge.

At Nombulelo's funeral, her daughter, Ntombizanele, stood up and read the following poem to the mourners who had gathered at a sports center to say good-bye to her mother, yet another woman who had succumbed to HIV/AIDS. It was titled "Kevin—Be Encouraged":

When the problems are more
And the resources are less
And you don't think you can stand
One more test
Be encouraged.

You cross a number of streets
In Cape Town, Guguletu, etc.
And heal the poor souls that were not having hope
Be encouraged.

Know that there are women
Fighting and caring too
We are encouraged from knowing you
So be encouraged.

You are such a bright star
And I love the bright warrior for justice
The Holy Spirit is blessing you
You will go far.

You are a man of love, honour and dignity
I'm proud to know you!
And I want to introduce you to the Guguletu poor people
And government as an example of beauty in humanity
Fighting on the ground for our people.

Because you are a light of hope
That changed our lives
And will shine bright
In our souls forever
Be encouraged.

Thank U.

A twelve-year-old girl, reading those lines to hundreds of mourners at her mother's funeral. Yes, I was adequately thanked for providing food on occasion and for helping to pay for Nombulelo's funeral. That I could do for this one family.

Shortly before I left South Africa, I ran into Ntombizanele on the street in Guguletu. She gave me a handwritten letter from her and her siblings that read: "Our mother loved us 'till she died. Even where she is now, we know that she did love us, and we will always remember what she gave us. She gave us that mother's love. We need someone to love us as our mother did. Kevin, do something about our situation. We love you; you love us. Take us somewhere where they will love us."

"Take us somewhere where they will love us." That I could not do for this family, no matter how many times they may thank me for it.

On the day I left Cape Town, Ntombizanele was at the airport waiting for my taxi to pull up to the international departure terminal, along with about forty other people from Guguletu. I didn't notice the group initially. It was the taxi driver who saw a group of people wearing "HIV Positive" T-shirts and red AIDS ribbon pins who said, "It looks like you made some friends during your stay here." That was an understatement.

For the next ninety minutes my South African friends, nearly all of them living with HIV/AIDS, sang and danced outside the terminal. Other travelers took pictures of our party and videotaped the singing and dancing. Four men from Turkey joined in the celebration and asked if I would send copies of my photographs to them in Istanbul. People who often go to bed hungry at night gave me gifts.

One member of the HIV/AIDS support group took me aside. In all of the excitement of the moment, I forget now who it was. She was holding something in her hand. "My father always said," she began, "that every man needs a flashlight to light his way in life. My father is dead now, and I want you to have his flashlight to light your way." With

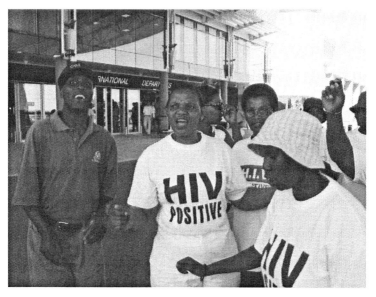

Departing Cape Town International Airport in 2004. The wind takes me to the United States, but the same wind keeps bringing me back to Guguletu.

that, she handed me a black flashlight, hugged me, and returned to the group, which continued to sing and dance.

Reverend Xapile, with whom I had worked so closely for over six months, approached me and said it was time for me to go. He was right. Members of the group were beginning to cry, and so was I. I crossed the street and before entering the terminal I turned to face the group one last time and yelled so that they all could hear me: "Enkosi kakhulu." Thank you very much.

When I returned to the United States, I had an e-mail from the Reverend waiting for me. In it, he explained what my well-wishers at the airport were saying to me in Xhosa that day I left South Africa: "Members of the support group were saying, 'Kevin is gone with the wind, but the same wind will bring him back.' "

His e-mail continued: "I know you will come back home. I will see you here at home. Our people are your people. Our home is your home. Our friends, your friends."

People who meant well had warned me that I would be taken advantage of in the townships of South Africa, that all people would want from me would be money, and that I would never be thanked for anything I did for them. "They will put out their hands, take whatever you give them, and that will be the end of the story."

Fortunately, the naysayers were wrong. That was not the end of the story.

EPILOGUE

♦
_____

A few days into the new year of 2004, I was walking down
a hospital corridor toward the room of a friend who was
dying, when I had a flashback. Just for a moment, it felt
like it was 1995 and I was in a hospital in upstate New
York, approaching the room of another friend who was
also dying. Of course it wasn't 1995. I wasn't in New York,
and I wasn't visiting my gay white friend who was dying
of AIDS. It was a new year in a new century. I was in Cape
Town, South Africa, and this time the friend dying of
AIDS was a black mother of three children.

My friends, John in the United States, and Nombulelo
in South Africa, could not have been more different. John
lived alone in his rambling, twelve-room house on the
Hudson River. Nombulelo lived in two small rooms in a
South African township with her aged mother, her children, a sister, and a nephew. John traveled the world and
ordered Dom Perignon as if it were water. Nombulelo
saw little of life outside of her township of Guguletu, and,
since she sometimes had to carry water from a public tap

_____

*Parts of this epilogue were first published in advocate.com on
March 16, 2004.*

to her home, she valued water more than the expensive champagne that John preferred. John hid his HIV status. The entire community knew Nombulelo had AIDS. After John died, he was cremated. There was no memorial service. For nearly two weeks after Nombulelo's death, the family held evening prayers in their tiny home. Hundreds of people came to her funeral, many wearing beaded red ribbon AIDS pins and "HIV Positive" T-shirts.

Two friends: a wealthy, white, gay man in America, and a poor, black mother in South Africa. The only thing they had in common was that they died of AIDS. Yet, when I think about Nombulelo, John creeps into my memory. And when I think about HIV/AIDS in South Africa today, more than twenty years into the pandemic, I'm transported back to the start of the AIDS epidemic in the U.S. in the 1980s. I keep asking the same question: don't we have a responsibility to help people living with HIV/AIDS wherever in the world they live?

For nearly ten years, I have had the privilege of being associated with Open Arms of Minnesota, a nonprofit organization based in Minneapolis, Minnesota. Bill Rowe, the curmudgeonly anthropology professor who founded Open Arms, believed he had a responsibility to help people living with HIV/AIDS in the Twin Cities of Minneapolis and St. Paul.

Bill had a passion for good food and nutrition. He also was a champion of those who could not advocate for themselves. In 1986, Bill realized that some of his acquaintances with HIV/AIDS were becoming too ill to shop for groceries and prepare meals for themselves. One evening he surprised a handful of those men by delivering a home-cooked meal to them. It was meant to be a single act of kindness, but the following week a few of the meal recipients called Bill to inquire if there would be another meal delivery. Bill said yes, and although he didn't know it at the time, Open Arms of Minnesota was born.

Since 1986, Open Arms has prepared and delivered more than one million meals to people—men, women, transgendered, straight, gay, bisexual, white, black, young, old—all living with HIV/AIDS, as well as their dependent children or affected caregivers. But Open Arms hasn't stopped there. The organization has continued to serve more and more people living with HIV/AIDS and in 2005 opened its arms wider to provide the same service— nutritious home-delivered meals—to women undergoing treatment for breast cancer and people with multiple sclerosis (MS) or amyotrophic lateral sclerosis (ALS).

In 2000, that small group of individuals from Open Arms, whom I accompanied on our first trip to South Africa, returned to Minneapolis and began talking about our global responsibility to assist people living with HIV/ AIDS half a world away. We couldn't figure out what to do. Well-intentioned people, who turned out to be wrong, cautioned us that any efforts we made to assist AIDS programs in Africa would only take resources away from our own community and Minnesotans living with HIV/AIDS. But we reasoned that if we could provide home-delivered meals to people living with HIV/AIDS in the Twin Cities, and there were people living with the same disease in a place like Guguletu who didn't have a thing to eat—I mean, not even a slice of bread—couldn't we do something for them? If most people with HIV/ AIDS in my state had access to the medications that would prolong their lives, and the most anyone we had met in Africa had to relieve the pain of end-stage AIDS was aspirin, wasn't there some way we could help? Didn't we at least have to try?

Six months after that initial trip I returned to South Africa with another group from Minnesota. Before traveling to Guguletu, we stopped in Johannesburg to visit a South African friend and AIDS pioneer, Nobesuthu Mnguni. Nobesuthu spent several days showing us the programs she was involved with and introducing us to even more people living with HIV/AIDS. One day, driving through Soweto, the huge township just outside of Johannesburg, Nobesuthu asked a simple question.

"Open Arms," she began. "What a beautiful name. Tell me, will Open Arms ever open its arms to Africa?"

That was a transformative moment for me. I knew I had to do something. I had spent enough time researching the pandemic and learning the statistics. I had been invited into the homes of South Africans who were living with, and dying from, the disease. In the future I could not say that I didn't know what was happening to millions of people with HIV/AIDS around the world. My very comfortable middle-class life in the United States could never be the same. I was now accountable.

Through Open Arms, we have tried to do our small part in assisting with global HIV/AIDS efforts. For our work to be successful in South Africa, we felt it was essential that any activities we sponsored there be closely aligned with the mission of Open Arms: "With open arms, we nourish body, mind and soul," and with our vision: "We see a world of abundance where people won't go hungry." We raise money to sponsor a hot lunch program for the members of the HIV/AIDS support group at the Zwane Community Centre in Guguletu. For approximately $75 a day, we can provide a hot lunch to any member of the support group or their affected family member who needs a meal. That amount pays for all of the food, the cook's salary, transportation to grocery stores and markets, kitchen supplies, and some general operating costs like gas and electricity.

We assembled and distributed our first food parcels on World AIDS Day in December 2003, and Open Arms now provides food parcels twice a year. Each parcel contains enough food to feed a family affected by HIV/AIDS for a month. The parcels overflow with rice, samp, oats, sugar, flour, tea, beans, canned fish, and vegetables. The groceries are placed in five-gallon plastic pails with lids. The pails make it easy for recipients to carry the food to their homes. They also give them something to store the food in to keep out bugs and rodents. When the food is gone, the pail can be used to fetch water from the public water taps.

Perhaps as important as the food itself is that Open Arm's partnership with the Zwane Community Centre in Guguletu gives us the opportunity to continually increase awareness of the global AIDS pandemic. We help remind Americans that HIV/AIDS is far from over and although it is a complex international challenge, there are simple things each of us can do to improve the lives of people living with HIV/AIDS in places in sub-Saharan Africa.

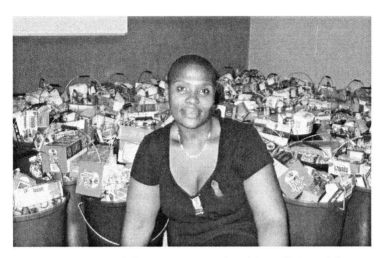

*Americans opened their arms to South Africans living with
HIV/AIDS by giving them food parcels.*

Part of our work is about putting a face on the global
AIDS pandemic—about getting Americans not to dwell
on the statistics but to see the impact this disease has on
one individual South African or on a particular South
African family. Open Arms had been doing this work for
several years—trying to get Americans to see and connect
with South Africans as individuals—before I realized that
we had been making no effort to have a similar impact on
South Africans' perceptions of Americans.

It's safe to say that for most South Africans, their impressions of the United States and Americans come from
the media, American entertainment (especially television
programs and movies), and our politics and international
policies. This is especially true in townships like Guguletu,
where most people have little substantive interaction with

whites and virtually no opportunities to meet Americans. How little we know each other struck home for me during a visit to South Africa in April of 2004.

I was driving from Guguletu to Cape Town at the end of an especially challenging day. My flight to South Africa from the States earlier in the week had been canceled, which resulted in my losing nearly two days of work in an already abbreviated trip. Then I came down with a violent case of food poisoning that kept me bed-bound for a day and left me physically weak for my remaining time in the country.

Although it's illegal to talk on a cell phone while driving in South Africa, on my way back to Cape Town that night I answered my ringing phone. It was a South African friend, who greeted me with a very terse question: "What has your country done now?"

I admit to being something of a news junkie in the States, but my time in South Africa is usually so jam-packed with activity that I end up in a current events void. I replied to my friend that I had no idea what he was talking about. He insisted I stop by an Internet café, sign on to a news site, and call him when I saw what he was referring to. I asked what I should look for on the site. How would I know what he was so upset about? "Believe me, you'll know the minute you're online," was his response.

I parked my car on the street and walked into the nearest Internet café I could find in Cape Town. I signed on to AOL and saw the image of a human figure, shrouded in a black poncho-like garment, a pointed black hood covering the head and face. The figure's arms were outstretched in what I thought initially must be some kind of an odd representation of a crucifixion. The next photo showed a man in an orange jumpsuit huddled on the floor, clearly cowering in front of a large German shepherd. By the third photo, a grinning American soldier with naked men piled up behind her, I had an idea of what my South African friend was referring to when he asked me what my country had done. The accompanying text confirmed that American soldiers had been torturing prisoners in an Iraqi prison none of us had ever heard of before called Abu Ghraib.

For my remaining days of that trip in South Africa, Abu Ghraib was all South Africans wanted to talk about. For some, it confirmed their long-standing suspicions about our government. They didn't want to discuss Abu Ghraib so much as they wanted to rail against all things American. I was working at the center in Guguletu when a member of the support group approached me to talk. He was troubled by the images of torture he had seen on television. "I thought Americans were the good guys," he said to me. I said I thought we were, too, but it was clear that the questioner was no longer sure.

This was yet another transformative moment in South Africa. I realized that through my work at Open Arms I had tried to get Americans to see that HIV/AIDS in Africa was about people, not statistics. I had spent no time, however, trying to get South Africans to see that not all Americans were like the characters on the hugely popular television series *Baywatch* and that not all Americans supported every aspect of our foreign policy. There had to be some way to build on the programs we were supporting in Guguletu so that they did more than just provide food and nutrition. We needed to find a way to start connecting individual South Africans with individual Americans who were sponsoring Open Arms' efforts in Guguletu. The food parcel program seemed like a logical place to start.

Members of the HIV/AIDS support group in Guguletu made a connection between the programs of Open Arms and me, since I was the face that they saw most often. It was time that they started to see, if not in person then, through pictures, the faces of other Americans who were concerned about their well-being. When I returned to the United States from that brief, politically charged trip, we added a component to our food parcel sponsorship.

We asked our American donors to contribute $35 to purchase all of the food and the plastic bucket that we needed for each food parcel. Then we asked them for more: to also give us a photo of themselves, or their family, or a loved one they wanted to recognize or remember. In a sentence or two, we told them to tell the person who would receive the food parcel in South Africa something about themselves or the person in the picture. We asked them to briefly tell the recipient why they were motivated to provide food to someone in Africa whom they would never meet.

The staff at Open Arms scanned each photograph onto a sheet of paper, along with the description of the donor and their motivation for helping someone with HIV/AIDS in Guguletu. We included a picture of the South African and the U.S. flags so that even South African recipients who didn't read English or were illiterate would make a visual connection between our two countries, and could probably deduce that their food parcel had come from the Americans pictured on the form that adorned their parcel.

Our efforts and gestures, I know, are small. For some people with HIV/AIDS in South Africa, Open Arms temporarily fills their stomachs with one meal a day. For others, the food parcel provides nourishment for a month or more. Some have told us that knowing that strangers in the United States care about people in South Africa is important to them. I have walked into a shack in Guguletu

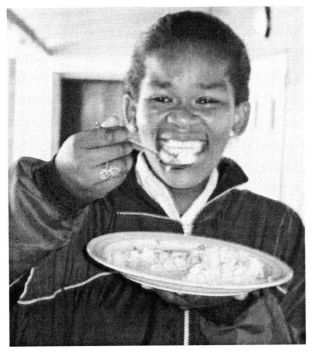

For less than a dollar a day, Open Arms can provide a hot lunch for people living with HIV/AIDS and their affected family members in Guguletu.

and seen a food parcel form proudly displayed on the wall of its recipient.

Will our efforts in Guguletu have any long-term effect on the people we serve there? Will the little food we provide improve the quality of their lives or ideally extend their lives? The next time the world is outraged by American foreign policy, will a few people in Guguletu better understand, because they received a food parcel, that Americans and American foreign policy are not always synonymous?

I don't know.

All I know is that I have lost too much and learned too much and gained too much—in the now twenty-five years of the AIDS pandemic—to ever give up. Those of us who have been touched by HIV/AIDS in this country have an opportunity to open our arms to others living with the same disease throughout the world. We can show the world how compassionate and generous Americans can be. And by doing this, we just may discover that people like my wealthy, gay, white friend John in New York, and my poor, straight black friend Nombulelo in South Africa, really weren't that different from each other after all.